Pretzel On Prozac

The Story of an Immigrant Dog

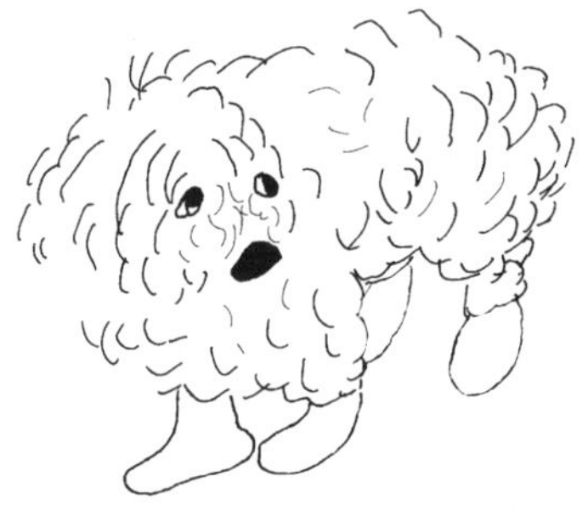

Other books by Ellen Palestrant

Nosedive
Johannesburg One Hundred
Remembering Dolores (co-editor)
I Touched A Star In My Dream Last Night
Have You Ever Had a Hunch? The Importance of Creative Thinking
The World of Glimpse
If You Can Make It, Mr. Harris...So Can I
If You Can Make It, Mr. Harris...So Can I: Teacher's Guide & Workbook

Pretzel On Prozac

The Story of an Immigrant Dog

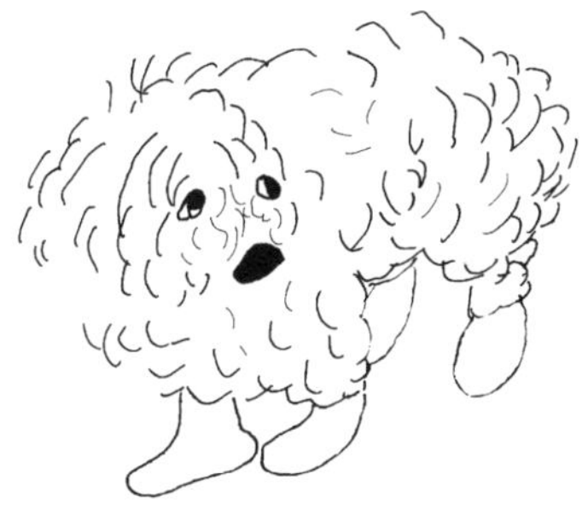

Ellen Palestrant

epCreative Enterprises

Pretzel on Prozac: The Story of an Immigrant Dog

First edition
2014 Printing

ISBN 978-0-9848852-2-0

Published by epCreative Enterprises

Cover and interior design: The Printed Page

Categories: Animal/Memoir/Literature/Psychology/Immigration

Printed in The United States of America

An Autobiodography

To the memory of Nathan—my beloved Nos.
Forever inspired by your curiosity and wisdom.
Forever in my heart.

Small dogs often live for fourteen, fifteen, or even sixteen years, but Pretzel lived to twenty. I would like to thank Dr. Chris Visser, veterinarian extraordinaire, and his dedicated staff for contributing to Pretzel's longevity.

Contents

When?

Eight in our family: N and I, our two sons, three dogs and a cat. Smokey, our cat, his grey coat flowing like dispensing hair mousse, always looks windswept. He is fifteen years old. So is our retiree Labrador Retriever, Omri. Black-coated, once shiny, once streamlined, once perfectly pectoraled and abdominaled, he is now, according to our vet, obese.

Insensitive usurpers, two toddler pups, have taken over: Haig, also a black Labrador, is plump and puckered. He is only eight weeks, while Bailey, a mop of a Maltese skimming the floor as he follows Haig, me, or anyone in his tasseled vision, is six weeks.

Bailey is the first Maltese we've ever had. He's alert, playful, cuddly, fearless and already has eight weeks worth of attitude in his jaunty gait. With head erect, long, silky-haired tail arched over his back, he swaggers and struts. When I pick him up and gaze into his wide-apart, inquisitive, black eyes, I'm melted.

"I'm putty in his paws," I say to N. "Let's get another Maltese."

Our sons agree. So does N even though we're making this decision to add a ninth member to our family at the same time we're discussing **when** to emigrate from South Africa to the United States: before or after our sons complete school.

"After," N says. "In time for college."

"Before," I say. "Best to get into the school system, sooner."

Each debate has merit. Apartheid doesn't. It's indefensible. We feel guilty for having been born into a country that adheres to a system of separating groups according to race. We know we must leave.

"When?" ask our sons.

Cocktails In Johannesburg

N and I visit a Maltese breeder who shows us the current litter of five. One pup stands out because he has a ginger ear, and because, with shrill indignation and an apparent sense of moral rectitude, he takes issue with us. *How dare you stare at me*, he babble-barks. We choose him.

"What shall we call him?" I ask N as we drive home with our new dog and his pedigree papers.

Smokey was the unremarkable name we'd given our cat, which prefers answering to "kssss-kssss-ksssssssss." Omri, inspired by the biblical King Omri of Israel, suits our stately, black, old Labrador. Our two pups are named after alcoholic beverages: Haig after *Dimple Haig* of dimpled bottle fame (my father's favorite—the contents—not the bottle) and Bailey, after my drink of choice, *Bailey's Irish Cream*, fifty percent triple distilled Irish whiskey and fifty-percent cream. Poured over vanilla ice cream, Bailey's is deliciously sickening.

"How about calling him Witblits?" suggests N.

"Witblits—white lightning." I liked the idea of naming him after home-distilled dop brandy. "Moonshine's nice, too."

"Mampoer?"

"Peach brandy—no."

"Maybe we need a name to accompany the drinks," says N.

"Biltong."

"Salami."

"Snacks."

We decide on *Pretzel*. He's not much bigger than one and his right ear is a glossy, ginger-golden, the color and sheen of salted pretzels.

Pedigrees: A First Encounter

I had never given pedigrees much thought until living with Omri, a perfectly proportioned, incorrigibly destructive of shoes, trees, plants, and toys (until the age of five), thoroughbred Labrador Retriever. An extremely handsome dog.

In his prime, his neck, muscular and free from throatiness, conformed to the desirable general appearance of his breed. So did his topline: horizontal from the withers to the croup. He was close to perfect: his teeth—strong and well-aligned; his tail—ample at the base, tapering proportionally to the tip; his nose—retrousse, black and wide; his nostrils—defined, flared, well-aired. His eyes—beaming adoration and loyalty.

"Beautiful," people would say of him.

"Should enter him in shows," a few suggested.

"Highly intelligent and impeccably *pedigreed,*" we added.

Remembering Pepsi

Now we have four pedigreed dogs—all beautiful—all loving. Yet the canines in my life before Omri had been mongrels, and just as intelligent. Ad hoc dogs with haphazard combinations of physical features and personalities: squat or willowy, rotund or puny, short-or-long-legged bodies with coats of black, brown, tan, grey and white, splashed, attached, and combined—any which way; unpredictable pets with faithful or disloyal intentions: stay-at-homers or get-up-and-goers, two-timers, three-and-more-timers. Philanderers. The would-abandon-you-for-a-bone type, even if the bone was years old with barely an aromatic trace of Eau de Boeuf or Leg d'Agneau Number Five.

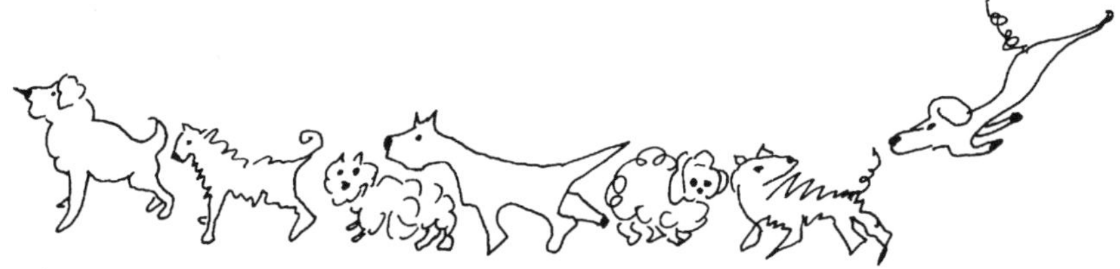

Take Pepsi, the dog-love of my childhood, so tiny he could fit into our mailbox—but not through the slot—couldn't slot him; so charmingly sociable that he wrapped people around the tip of his wagging, furry tail. He magnetized many middle-class people in our neighborhood (who lived in lines of twenty-feet-from-the-sidewalk, red-roofed houses) towards his demands; enthralled them with his hungry, hopeful, beseeching eyes:

"Hey, Pepsi, want a meatball?" He would be fed home-cooked, warmed-up, human food—yesterday's meatball-frikkadel, drowning in grease, or a curried sosatie.

"Want some bones?" That night's braai beef ribs.

"Mince meat?" Curried bobotie—baked in the oven with apricots and almonds—prepared in advance for tomorrow.

"Boerewors?" Especially fryed for him as he waited.

Pepsi knew what he wanted and would go to great lengths to satisfy his needs. If he wished to visit my married sister, he would walk to her apartment complex—a few blocks from our house—climb up the stairs to the second floor, and if she wasn't in, tap on the doors of her friends on the first and third floors—in that order—hoping to find her.

"Is she here? Yes! Got you! Private-Eye Pepsi does it again."

If he needed my company of a morning, he would visit my school and pester the stodgy staff until they caved in and sent someone to find me. I was especially pleased if this happened during a history lesson, which it often did. Pepsi seemed to enjoy interrupting the teacher's themes:

"Jislaaik, you can't let whites be overwhelmed!"

"Domkops, don't you know whites came to South Africa long before the natives?"

Wrong, black migration preceded white migration. You think we don't have discussions at home? My internal dialogue is then halted by a knock on the door: Pepsi and the school secretary.

"Again!" shouts the teacher. "Take your blerrie dog home!"

"Sorry."

As I leave the classroom with Pepsi and proceed along the corridor, I can still hear him:

"God wants nations and people to be separate."

And teachers and pupils. I'm immensely grateful to my dog, and repeatedly tell him so as I carry him home. After making sure the gates are closed, I stroll back to school. A gift of a free hour!

An Independent Thinker

Pepsi was so defiant that he never obeyed anything resembling an order:

All rules are to be challenged.

Most are obsolete and do not in any way relate to my present situation.

Independent Pepsi, on any given cue, let you know that he didn't need you and that he didn't need to be bound by any societal definition of canine behavior. Did as he pleased. From the beginning, Pepsi demanded of us that we never be straight-forward with him, never hinder his freedom, always let him overrule rules and make his own.

"Out! Out! Out, Pepsi!"

To entice him indoors at night, my mother and I had to pretend that we wanted him outdoors or that his existence was as unnoticeable to us as a quark in the dark. Then, when he was quite sure we were completely unaware of him, he'd demand our attention by tearing into the house while barking loudly, ready now to curl up on his rug and go to sleep. This was just what we'd wanted from him in the first place, but hadn't dared to suggest because always, Pepsi had to establish that this was *his* choice, not ours. He had trained us well.

Did the fact that Pepsi was a mongrel account for his independent, idiosyncratic, and unpredictable attitude? Not sure if having a pedigree brings out the best in a dog and dictates more dependable behavior—a living-up-to-your-label thing. Never been dazzled by titles. Always felt that a dependency on family trees, designer labels, and on the broadcast of one's accomplishments which fit into a current CATALOG OF PERCEIVED SUCCESS, are signs of weakness, emphasizing a lack of, rather than an abundance of confidence and ability. An unstudied, serendipitous self-evolvement, I think, is more interesting than a definable, socially-agreed-upon, self-involvement.

So why now, do we have four pedigreed dogs?

Pedigreed Pretzel

"Some lineage!" I examine our new Maltese's pedigree. Hate to say that I'm impressed. How can I be so hypocritical? Actually like the fact Pretzel has a posh pedigree, even more august than our other thoroughbreds. Real blue blood connections. Pretzel is the closest I've ever come to living with royalty. I have great expectations of him and he has much to live up to. So, perhaps, have I.

According to his *Certificate of Pedigree* and his *Certificate of Transfer* from the Kennel Union of South Africa, he comes from aristocracy—from a recognized breed served by a registry—from a really good family. He was born to Sigmasix Donald and Sigmasix Dynamite whose great great great-grandsire and great great great-grandam, Vic Snippet of Frantoit and Elisa Snod of Fremantle were imported into South Africa from the United Kingdom.

"Looks like Pretzel is descended from the British Upper Class," I tell N. "From inherited wealth, from dogs that didn't have to work for a living."

"Or clean their own kennels," says N.

I compare Haig and Bailey's papers.

"Haig's papers, like Pretzel's, are accompanied by a *Certificate of Transfer*," I tell N. "Bailey's aren't. The breeder said she didn't have one, when we asked."

"Maybe Bailey's papers aren't authentic," says N.

"You think that his bloodline doesn't go back to Great Grand Sire Kooki Kooks Von Kikooki and Great Grand Dam Mitzie Des Abois as it states here?"

But really, who cares. Bailey *looks* like a Maltese—almost. His temperament reminds me of Pepsi's. I don't mind if Bailey is an impersonator. He is his own dog. Status doesn't define him. Intelligence does. Experiencing freedom, he runs around the house and garden without waiting for Haig or Pretzel to follow him. When he needs boundaries, he appoints me his shepherd. Follows me wherever I go. I'm touched by his dependence. I have a little lamb.

Tales About Tails: A Dog's

Funny—no, actually it's not funny having three pups of under ten weeks old to be socialized and potty-trained at the same time, each with different temperaments, learning abilities, and varying needs. Haig and Bailey are assertive. They vie for our attention, letting us know what they want, but Pretzel is undemanding. Doesn't learn as quickly as the others. Some resistance here.

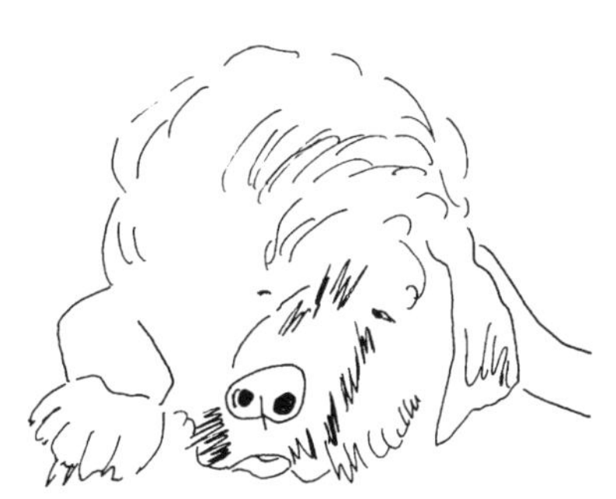

Omri sleeps most of the time. Lies on his stomach while the pups, captained by Bailey, a natural leader, play with his heavy, unresisting tail, swinging it from side to side, and pulling at its tapered tip—a Tug Of War—trying to drag the black, furry rope across an imaginary line:

"One, two three—PUUUlllllllllllllllllllllllllllllllllll!!!!!!!! "

Omri doesn't seem to notice or mind the pups tugging his tail. His mind is far away from his tired, arthritic body. Sadly, their playfulness fails to invigorate him. The *Omri Team* never budges. Keeps its equilibrium. Wins—

tail-down. The *Barely-out-of-Diapers Team* always loses, but the members' tails wag happily as Omri sleeps on.

Tales About Tails: A Cat's

Smokey is unimpressed with the pups. With feline disdain, he ignores them and keeps his distance, hissing and arching his back if they approach. Spends most of his time in his favorite place—on a comfortably padded dining room chair. Smokey doesn't have a tail: One night, in shock and covered in blood, he leapt through an open window into our sitting room with only a thin, long caudal vertebrae attached to his behind. We wrapped him in a towel and rushed him to an emergency veterinary surgery where the remaining vestige of his once noble rear guard was amputated. The following morning, we found his thick, furry tail on our patio. He'd been skinned. Still don't know what happened.

Smokey took time to adjust to having a stump instead of a beautiful, long, flexible tail to aid his balance. Without this extension of himself which he had habitually straightened when he spotted potential prey, and twitched—tip-tail—when angry, he had lost an important part of his self-expression and communication. Even worse, he had lost his stability and now lacked counterbalance. Without his tail, so integral a part of himself, Smokey underwent a change of identity. Became a guinea pig in some failed laboratory experiment.

Omri, Haig, Bailey, and Pretzel need their tails and so did he. So do horses, giraffes, lions, leopards, mink, raccoons—the list goes on. But humans survive with a suggestion of a tail at the base of their spines and Manx cats from the Isle of Man, do perfectly well without theirs. Schipperke, bred in Belgium to be watchdogs on boats, and Barbary apes, found in Algeria, Morocco and Gibraltar, manage well without tails. Indri, echidna, koalas and wombats don't particularly yearn for their tails. Eventually, nor did Smokey.

But for a while, he needed his tail:

"So embarrassing!" He fell off the kitchen counter. Landed on his feet.

"Utterly mortifying!" After walking along our rooftop, he was unable to come down. Too scared.

Smokey had lost his tail and his feeling of invulnerability. The encouraging *Ksss-kssss-kssssssssssss* from all of us didn't help. N had to climb up to rescue him. Smokey didn't purr or trill for days. But about two weeks after his surgery, he regained his equilibrium—and his dignity.

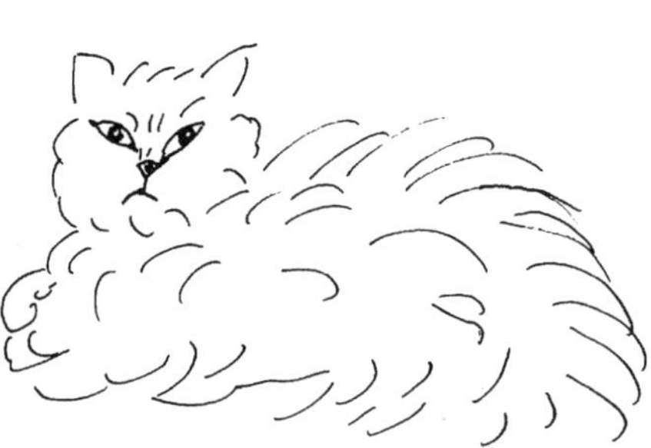

Goodbye Omri

Omri died of kidney failure. We'd known that he didn't have long to live, but were shocked to find him inert, terminally still, lying on his stomach—his usual position—his tail now a heavy dead-weight. The athletic pup and teenage dog that had pulled out fruit trees as soon as they were planted, again and again when we planted more, leaving us guessing whether the surviving trees would bare plums, apricots or peaches, was no more. The shiny, densely-coated delinquent, who had pulverized our shoes and anything else he could grip between his teeth, and the regal adult dog with an appetite so voracious that he took to eating newspapers when the vet advised us to drastically reduce his food intake, was gone. Fifteen years old. He'd had a long life, and in the end dwelled more frequently outside his body than in it. But now his re-entry visa has expired. We're going to miss him. Greatly.

Bailey, Haig and Pretzel haven't noticed his absence. I think he was just a tail to them.

The Art of Sailboarding

Bailey is fearless. Leaps from boulders with the nonchalant, suspended-in-animation-look of an experienced skydiver. Loves water. Goes up and down our swimming pool on a surfboard. Loves boats: sailboats, ski-boats, dinghies, dories. Loves water sports of any kind.

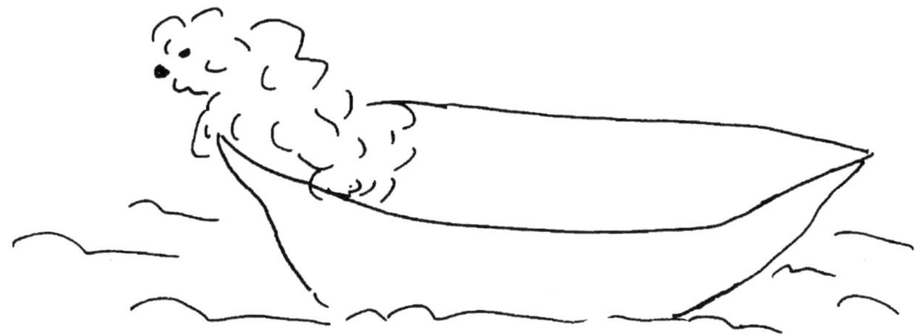

We took Bailey sailboarding on Hartebeestpoort Dam last Sunday. Intrepid little dog. A white fleck sailing for the perilous unknown on a vast waterway beneath the Magaliesberg Mountains. A dot of a dog with his snout to the south, resolutely never looking back.

Bailey is a natural. Fell off the board a couple of times but was happy to swim in that thick, pea-green, water--hyacinth-infested, oxygen-depleted soup until we helped him onto the board again. Haig sails too. Both have the right sailing stance. Both have co-ordinated swimming strokes and professional attitudes. They didn't need lessons or life jackets. Upwind, downwind, headwind, tailwind, it didn't matter to them. They adapted their carriage, transitioning their paws on the board—freestyle—their very own style, according to the prevailing winds. Nonchalantly, they mastered the art of sailboarding and, eventually, re-boarding when they fell into the water. Cool dogs.

Not A Water Dog

Pretzel's never cool. We had assumed that he would be more like Bailey, but he isn't. Puzzling, since they are both Maltese. We've tried to put him on a sailboard, took him sailing, attempted to teach him to swim in our pool, coaxed him to jump into puddles, but he'll have none of this. Hates water. Squeals in anguish when sprayed by our sprinkling system. Nothing will induce him to wet his silky curls. Not even for all the wedges of a Cadbury's chocolate bar will he place one paw in a puddle. Nor for all the biltong in South Africa will he wet his round, black snout. Not even to gain the respect of Bailey and Haig will he suppress his yelps when he is bathed. He prefers to watch them being shampooed, or splashing and muddying themselves in the garden after it's rained.

Haig and Bailey log up their weekly miles in our pool. Pretzel runs around the perimeter, barking happily as they dog-paddle their laps—many times a day. They ignore him. Afraidy-Dog. Chicken. They've dismissed him.

Bailey tolerates Pretzel and bullies Haig—the mate with which he chooses to hobnob but the one he continually chides. They dash around our garden together, barking at visitors, at imaginary intruders, and at each other. Bailey tries to keep up with the effortless sprint of Haig around our half-acre garden, but his short legs fail him. Poor bandy Bailey. They both chase birds and balls, and Pretzel chases them in confused bliss, often looking back at us to see if we notice how happy he is, how much fun he is having. Sometimes he seems to beseech them, "Just *notice* me," but Bailey and Haig have disenfranchised him. He is not relevant to their lives, but they are to his. Especially Bailey.

Goodbye Smokey

Smokey died today. Suffered all weekend. Wish we'd put him down on Friday. Hadn't realized how ill he was. Thought he might improve. Kidney failure. He was seventeen.

Smokey had eventually accepted the new dogs. Just as he and Omri would sleep in our living room on their backs, bellies exposed, he started doing the same with Bailey and Haig—all three of them, belly up, secure in our protective custody. But not Pretzel. He slept belly down because somewhere the Bogey Dog lurked, ready to drench him with water.

Smokey sometimes slept with Pretzel. Never saw Smokey hiss at him as he did with the others. Pretzel was as unthreatening to him as a kitten.

Pangs Of Remorse

July One—next week—we're immigrating to the United States. All of us: N and me, our two sons—in time to start college, two of our dogs—Pretzel and Bailey.

It's hard to leave Haig behind, but there's no guarantee we'll have a garden big enough for him, and Labradors need roaming space. Gave him to a friend a few months ago—a dog lover with lots of acreage, leaving ourselves enough time before we depart to find him another home, should this one not work out. It has. Haig has settled down well. He is taken boating and fishing. Leads both a domestic and a rugged, out-of-doors' life. Sleeps under my friend's bed at night. She says he snores, but she doesn't mind. Says he's intelligent. Affectionate. An ideal dog.

We often park our car outside Haig's new home so that we can watch him play in the garden with the children, both under five. He runs after them, up and down the big expanse of lawn, undoubtedly enjoying himself. He's happy; we're guilty. Pangs of remorse surface unbidden. Can't forget his face pressed against the steel bars of the gate, perplexed that we were driving off without him.

Bailey adjusted quickly to Haig's absence and bullies Pretzel instead, yet they're mates and sleep together now. Pretzel understands that Bailey is boss and doesn't attempt to assert himself.

Sometimes I see Smokey asleep on our dining room chair. How our habits influence perceptions. Will I still see him asleep on the same chair when it's in a different room in another place, a foreign space in America? I miss him. I miss Omri, and I miss Haig. Living in the United States is not Haig's destiny, nor that of many of the people we leave behind.

So many goodbyes. So much we'll miss.

Immigrant Furniture

Our furniture left yesterday. Bubble-wrapped memories shipped to our future: giant, fragrant sachets of embalmed dissolving compounds of our past—of Africa, cradle of our beings; handspun and handwoven mohair tapestries from Namibia, wool rugs from Botswana, Bophutha Tswana, Swaziland; beaten copper, sandstone, soapstone, ironwood, yellowwood, and Msimbiti wood carvings from Zimbabwe, Zambia, and Kwazulu; paintings of Johannesburg—skyscrapers and shebeens; sketches of the bare bundu—the hot, dry Great Karoo—dolerite hillocks, thatched-domed rondavels, herds of Merino and Dorper sheep.

A passerby who looked like an inspector—of what I don't know—stopped to watch the movers load into a container our beds, sofas, tables, paintings, boxes of books and photographs powdered with the fine dust of the city. Dust to dust; Johannesburg to Phoenix.

"Are you immigrating?" he asked me.

"No, only our furniture," I replied. He looked at me strangely. How paranoid we are in South Africa, I thought. How secretive.

Immigrant Dogs

Today Pretzel and Bailey were crated for export. After first being tranquilized by the Pet-to-Jet's dognapper, they dozily and trustingly followed our reassuringly familiar, worn—especially-not-washed-for-this-occasion socks into a cage parked on our lounge carpet.

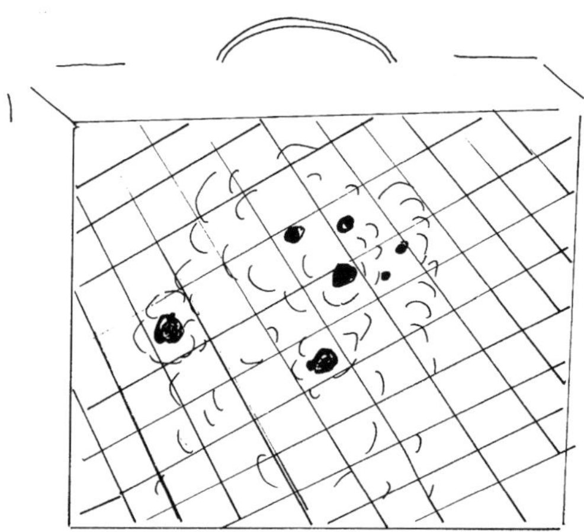

"See you in Arizona," we said as they were placed into the back of a van parked in our driveway. Inside, there were other incarcerated, narcotized emigrants—dogs, cats, birds, fish, ticks, and fleas, bound for Jan Smuts Airport, Johannesburg, and then to foreign destinations.

Reality. No turning back. It's our turn tomorrow. Excited, apprehensive, optimistic, and sad, very sad, we bid our farewells: Goodbye family. Goodbye friends. Goodbye Times Past—good times and bad times. Fair to middling times. Goodbye house, garden, street, neighborhood, Johannesburg—dynamic city of wealth, innovation, despair and danger; city of gold, of modern, streamlined high rises above pavements strewn with hopelessness and litter. Goodbye highveldt with its rocky koppies and tall, dry, yellow winter grass. Goodbye South Africa. We'll miss you. Totsiens.

Two Live Dogs

Bailey and Pretzel reached Phoenix the day before we did. Family, already living in the city, picked them up at Sky Harbor Airport. Took them to their apartment, but, when they released them from the crate which they'd placed on the kitchen counter, the jet-lagged, canine immigrants immediately marked their territory—days' worth of urine on the counter-top. Then they jumped and jumped and jumped and continued jumping the next day when we arrived. They were trying to tell us they'd been flying.

I examined their crate which had later been placed on the balcony. Our socks, which had substituted for us, were still inside. They could now be discarded. The crate was clearly addressed to our temporary residence in Phoenix, Arizona. The Air Waybill stated: "The goods described herein are accepted in apparent good order and condition for carriage." The Shipper's Certification had entered on its form under "Species": TWO LIVE DOGS.

Little did Bailey and Pretzel know what lay ahead for them when they left their Johannesburg home. From all accounts, the trip to the United States was frightening—even for a confident Top Dog, certainly for an apprehensive Under Dog. Although their accommodation was roomy, Bailey, demanding as usual most of the space for himself, probably compressed Pretzel into a corner. Sat on him, too. Pretzel looked shorter—flatter than he had in Johannesburg. Squashed.

Two live dogs indeed! How live could they have felt from the time they left a wintry South Africa as cargo aboard the KLM Royal Dutch Airlines and flew across continents and oceans, via Amsterdam, to Los Angeles, their point of entry into the United States where they were examined for evidence of contagious diseases, asked if they'd ever been members of the Communist Party, been subversive, insurrectional or perfidious—or if their owners had.

With a clean bill of physical and political health and much burbling in their bellies (hadn't eaten since South Africa), their emotional well-being was further impaired when their crate was misplaced at LAX airport before finally arriving in Phoenix. These two live dogs desperately in need of a potty, these two live dogs checked as baggage against their own volition, had immigrated into an oven of our choosing—115 degrees in the shade. Two hot dogs.

East Of West

Scottsdale: "The West's most Western Town." Just east of Phoenix. Been here for four months. Moved three times. Settling into dislocation. Can't find my way around the city without first consulting a map. Floundering. Groping for direction in new territory and ad-libbing for a living. Immigration is all about re-creation—about rethinking, remolding and repackaging yourself, but, at the same time, keeping your integrity. A tall order.

Pretzel embodies an immigrant's fears. He has become increasingly suspicious of anything new, quakes at the slightest noise. I worry about him and mentally instruct him: *Be receptive to new ideas, Pretzel. Transcend boundaries. Try this new doggie biscuit.* ***Don't*** *look the other way so that you can't see it. It can still see you. Won't hurt you. Has flaxseed and whey in it. It's good for you. Folic acid and vitamin B supplement, too. So taste America. Venture into unchartered territories. No time for preconceived notions. You're only five years old. Lots still to learn. Be open to the new. Opportunities abound.* When I address him this way, I rehearse for my future in America, for important discussions, for unverbalized areas of longings.

"How long will it take me to understand America?" I ask aloud.

Who am I in America anyway? One among many hopeful smidgens in this great composite of almost every nation on earth. *You've immigrated to the Land of Generosity, Pretzel, to a giant bottomless coffee pot, with second, third and tenth cups of coffee free. Now, how many countries offer that? At the airport in Rome, I had to pay for the milk and sugar added to my coffee in addition to the cup of stale beverage. There are so many ways to live your life in the USA. So many choices. You can be any dog you wish. Remember, you have a pedigree. Live up to your label. Wear it or change it. Don't look back. Don't be scared. Just look at Bailey.*

Bailey embraces choice. The unknown is exciting for him. Appreciatively, he gulps down new food, nonchalantly, he urinates against unfamiliar trees, and wickedly, despite our admonitions, he attacks the ankles of strangers. So many new blends of compounds to sniff, isolate, compare, play with, and reject. The essence of the United States, he believes, is contained in ankles, and the more snapshots he gets, the more he captures it.

The essence of America, I believe, is contained in the vast assortment of its affordable coffee beans selected from around the world: caffeinated, decaffeinated, ground or whole, blended, brewed, French-pressed, autodripped, cappuccinoed, and espressoed into distinctive tastes—for the purists and the perfunctory alike, for the rich and the poor. What's available in other countries is available here because immigrant beans, following other immigrant beans, settle down well in the States and continue to awaken the public to what's brewing—the aroma of the new.

Bailey doesn't need coffee to awaken him. Alert to the slightest hint of an opportunity, this self-directed dog is always focused. He attempts anything that **he** chooses and has never appeared resentful of the fact that we didn't ask his permission to fly him to the United States, and that we tricked him into immigration by proffering drugs and socks. I suspect that had we asked him, he would probably have made a ja-yeh, instant decision to transition. *Why not? Always land on my feet. I'm Top Dog.*

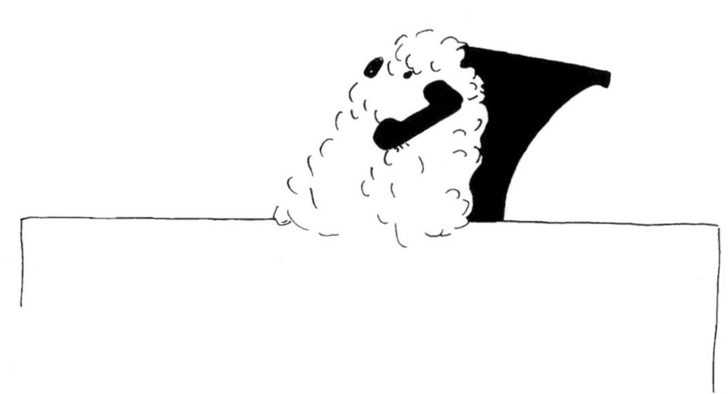

Unsettled In Scottsdale

Pretzel hasn't settled well. Living in three locations in such a short time—actually four counting the airplane—may have contributed to his nervousness. He jumps at the slightest noise. Is becoming increasingly distrustful of anything new. Needs a lot of reassurance.

Not only is the accommodation unfamiliar to him, but so is the vegetation. The first time Pretzel raised his back leg to urinate against a Saguaro, that great symbol of the American Southwest, he no doubt was pricked on the most delicate part of his under-belly. An assault by an assegai. Traumatic for a little dog that had previously been secure with the vegetation in his Johannesburg garden: the twice-weekly-mown kikuyu grass, eucalyptus, acacia and mimosa trees, with branches too tall to snare him; shrubs too good natured to stab or trip him, and rockeries overgrown with protea and prickly pear, in peripheral areas he knew to avoid.

Inescapable in Johannesburg, but known to him and therefore not feared, were the spear-happy khakiweed and blackjack growing along the sidewalks which would attach to his thick coat. Revolting were the hideous Parktown Prawns, two-inch King Crickets populating the garden, defecating vile-smelling black faeces when disturbed. I never saw Pretzel sniff or stalk one of these. Once, after putting on my pantyhose, I found a live one entrapped, and it relieved itself on my leg—noxious black effluvium—two hundred million years in evolution. The mere thought of that creature still evokes the shock and disgust I felt at the time. Ever since, I have remained hyper-vigilant to resident crickets in my hose.

Forget the past, Pretzel. Embark on new adventures. Fear is understandable but don't become immobilized by uncertainty. Don't be scared of new alternatives. No Parktown Prawns here to defecate on your spirits. Lots of scorpions, though. Don't be fearful, Pretzel. Not everything is controllable. Simply adjust to the fact that although coyotes, hawks and owls might think you are a fluffy white mouse and eat you up, they probably won't even notice you.

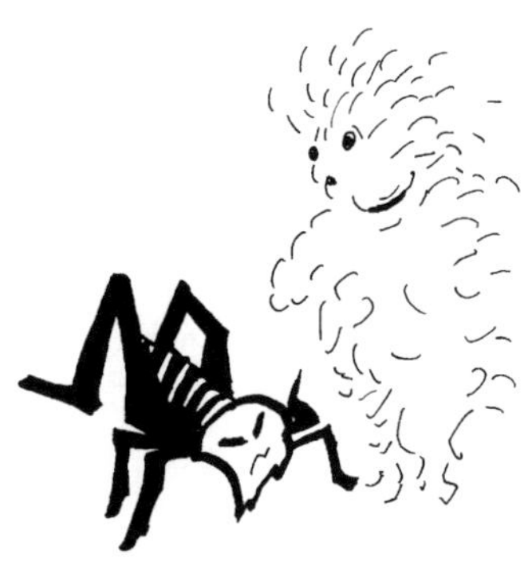

Puzzling Over Pretzel

Pretzel doesn't adapt. A routine-bound dog, not open to change, he has difficulty internalizing unfamiliar experiences and transferring from one situation to another because he learns little. Has a set amount of repertoires from which he draws and that's it. He barely amends these or adds to them. Pretzel, glued to his neuroses, is poor immigrant material as he still lives in a past that wasn't that vast.

Pretzel, accept change. Look, if your old government can finally reinvent itself, so can you. Apartheid is on the road to extinction. Restrictions on opposition groups have been lifted. Nelson Mandela has been released after twenty-seven years in prison. There is no longer a State of Emergency.

Three years in America, and Pretzel's state is one of constant emergency. Doom looms, and therefore, he remains distrustful of his environment, of anything new. Take the doggie door, for example: He fears its flap and won't approach it. What does he think? That it will deliver a knockout punch, reel him backwards, leave him flat on his back, flatter than the flap?

As the plastic flap swings both ways—towards the inside and outside of the house, we've placed roast beef—his favorite—just inside and outside the flap, but

Pretzel will not push it to exit or enter the house. He freezes. Closed doors remain closed doors.

So we have to keep the doggie door permanently open for Pretzel—and for all the mosquitos, cockroaches, crickets, spiders, and scorpions wishing to enter our house. Because we allow in the hot air in summer and the cold in winter, we can't conserve energy. Instead, we increase the load on the heating and cooling systems and on our bank account.

What would make Pretzel into a successful immigrant? The same qualities required of any newcomer: a desire to be challenged by the unfamiliar. Receptivity to new experiences. Suspension of criticism until a deeper insight is gained into the complexities of a new land, and desistance from comparisons with the old. An ability to bend, harmonize, and diverge, while finding a way into the constantly evolving reality of the present.

So Pretzel, what would make you into a good immigrant? Okay, for a start, simply press your nose against the flap of the doggie door and create an opening.

Salad Bar

Bailey loves sweet green peas—sugar peas, snap peas, petit pois—fresh or canned. Squints as he watches a hard, crunchy, uncooked pea roll across the tiled kitchen floor before stalking it, pouncing on it, and chewing it with the vigor given to a meat bone. Then, of course, he swallows it and searches for more. Gets frustrated when he drops a pea and it disappears beneath the refrigerator or dishwasher. Puts his snout next to the gap between the appliance and floor and snorts persistently, beseeching the pea to return.

We keep cans of young, tender peas in our pantry especially for Bailey. He loves food of any kind. Pretzel only likes meat, chicken, and chocolate. Both dogs are passionate about chocolate, especially chocolate kisses and chocolate chip cookies, but we've stopped giving those to them recently because we've learned that chocolate is bad for dogs. Never knew that. Reared our previous dogs on chocolate and they lived long, cacao-filled lives. Chocolate contains an ingredient called theobromine, which potentially is toxic to dogs. Can even be fatal.

We're scared now that even a lick of these bad slabs could result in an accumulative overdose because of all the theobromine which has already stock-piled in their constitutions. So we didn't wean them from their addiction. Just cut off their supply. Overnight, we stopped giving them Hershey kisses, Hershey Hugs and Hershey Nuggets to munch on while they watched television. Stopped giving them the chocolate chip cookies we'd especially selected for them and shared with them, replete with semi-sweet and very sweet, rich, milky morsels in crunchy, chompy, delicious, hydrogenated, triglycerided, real butter-and-egg crust that melted in their mouths. Poor dogs have gone cold turkey. So have we. At night they whine for chocolate; so do we.

Bailey is a glutton. No finesse. He eats everything. No problem selecting food for him. Pretzel is persnickety about what he eats and self-conscious about being watched while he does so. Something rather formal about him. Has his own idea about what is good form, and I suspect that if he were caught with crumbs on his chin or lettuce between his teeth, he would be embarrassed. Don't know what his problem with eating in public is. His table manners are just fine.

Pretzel tires quickly of dog food and has no attachment to any brand. So I give him choice. Give him the dilemma instead of me. Often I line up five bowls with different contents on our brick patio—like a salad bar. Then, after setting him down with his back to his food—a few yards away from the bowls because he always bolts in the opposite direction from the one he faces—I leave him to his usual ritual: approach food, withdraw, advance, recoil, inch-and-flinch—forward-backward, circle the patio neurotically, compulsively, before, finally, with body squared over whichever bowl beckons, ravenously demolish the contents.

The danger of this lengthy procedure is that if Bailey hasn't eaten first, or has but he isn't sated (Pretzel usually lets Bailey eat first—his response to Bailey's sense of entitlement), Bailey will gobble up Pretzel's food, leaving Pretzel dismayed over the emptiness of his bowls and his life. I then start the process all over again.

Hunger Strike

Bailey likes it when we have guests. Convinced they've come to visit him. Demands to be picked up so that he can look them in the face while they converse. High-level talks. Eye to eye. Man to dog.

Man: Are you *dog*matic?

Dog: Dogmatism is cowardly. I'm Bailey the Intrepid. I relish incertitude and ambiguity.

Man: What am I?

Dog: A guest.

Pretzel likes guests as long as they don't stay overnight, taking my attention away from him. If they unpack their belongings in the guest room, dismay overwhelms him. *I know it, I know it, I'm going to be sidelined,* ***again***! Can't disassociate himself from the foreboding he feels as underwear moves into drawers, and jackets drape garment hangers.

We have family visiting us for a few weeks. The parents sleep in the guest room and the two kids in my office. Once again, unfamiliar clothing hangs in the cupboard, and Pretzel has that *I'm-just-a-no-doggy* look. Defeated. Slumped. In the dumps.

"Do you think he doesn't want us to be here?" one of the kids asks. That's how obvious Pretzel is.

"Don't take it personally. Some previous guests have monopolized our attention and invaded Pretzel's space. Really, this has nothing to do with your visit. He keeps reliving the past. That's the kind of dog he is."

I don't want our guests to feel unwelcome, but Pretzel does. His mournful eyes, and forlorn body, tell us each time we look his way: *I am the outcast dog, the peripheral dog roaming the outskirts of my own home. No-one cares about me. Why don't you all leave?"*

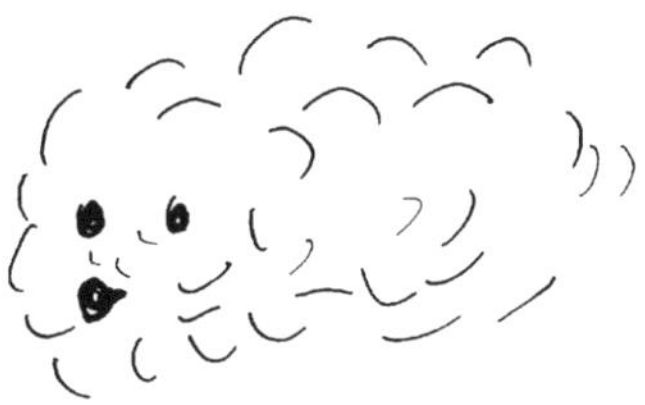

They don't. Pretzel refuses to eat or drink. Goes on a hunger strike. For days, he doesn't eat a morsel. Becomes weak. Sleeps all the time.

"He'll die if he doesn't at least drink," I tell N. "I'd better take him to the vet." So I sneak out of the house with Pretzel. I don't want our guests to feel guilty—but they do an hour later, when I have to explain his absence.

"Can't find Pretzel," the kids tell me as I enter the house. "We've looked all over for him."

"Took him to the vet because he wasn't eating," I tell them. "Will pick him up tomorrow. He's on a drip. Has to be fed intravenously."

"It's because of us," they all say.

"No, it's because of Pretzel."

For the remainder of their visit, I try every kind of delicious food I can think of to induce Pretzel to eat—

beef, lamb, liver, even a taste of chocolate—but Bailey consumes it all. We take Pretzel to the vet three more times to be fed intravenously. Next month, we're expecting more guests. What are we going to do with him?

Should We Take Them For A W-A-L-K?

By day or night, three hundred and sixty-five times a year we walk Pretzel and Bailey—whatever the weather. In the heat of summer we carry a water-filled plastic spray bottle—their personal misting and fogging system—for cooling them as they sniff and strut. When the sidewalks become stove-top hot, we put socks on their paws lest their soles fry. These help also in preventing burrs from sticking between their toes. In the relative-cool of Phoenix winter, we sprint around the lake together. Pretzel and Bailey demand these walks. Never allow us to forget them. Run around the house claiming our attention when they think it's time to go.

"Should we take them for a W-A-L-K?" We spell the word these days instead of saying it in Bailey's presence because merely articulating the word ignites a repetitive leapfrogging which can be alleviated only by rushing immediately out of the house with him and Pretzel.

Pretzel and Bailey regularly climb Camelback Mountain with us. Huffing and puffing inelegantly, Bailey stops at ledges to rest. He seems to contemplate the view below, selecting vantage points as if he knows what he wants to see:

Ah Scottsdale—can see the roof of my house! Ah Pinnacle Peak, the Four Peaks in the horizon, the MacDowells, Tempe, Paradise Valley, Phoenix.

When N and I reach the summit on clear days and admire the panoramic vista of the complete Valley of the Sun, or lament on smoggy days about the pollution robbing us of our view and our health, Bailey casually contemplates the grandeur, too. Then he looks back and down, triumphantly. He has completed the urban climb with us and with the other city dwellers he sees en route—some with dogs. How far he has come on his four, short, bandy legs! City Dog, the sociable climber, has reached the top and what a view!

Aaaahhhhhhhh.... I'm Top Dog.

Pretzel simply runs ahead. Doesn't look right nor left. Never assesses where he's going or from where he has come. Has no sense of his personal achievement or of the hardy doggedness it took to ascend steep, slippery conglomerate sandstone formations embedded with sharp rocks, granite boulders, and strewn with pebbles on which to slip and trip. He experiences the physical sensations of the moment and his body synchronizes with the elements, but he, modest dog, has no idea how athletic he looks as he leaps from one rock to the next.

Pretzel and Bailey sniff their way up the mountain, distinguishing one odor from another, however minute the molecular traces. With excitement, they identify the familiar track imbedded in their olfactory memories.

What do they see when they climb with their eyes so close to the ground? Vented, indented, blurry boots and sneakers? Sandy socks cushioning the jolts of uneven rocks? Do they ever see the purple and orange wild flowers growing next to the path? Do they glimpse the blue sky? Bailey might; not Pretzel.

Looking down or ahead, seldom sideways, Pretzel misses the surprising shapes of formations evolved over millions of years—a camel silhouette, a praying monk, or configurations of imaginations. He misses the chalky redness of the cliffs, the long shadows of saguaros, the cholla, agave, yucca, prickly pear, jojoba, palo verde, and mesquite trees. Yesterday, Pretzel missed identifying the jumping cholla—mean plant. It loosened its spiny joints against him when he brushed against it, and he objected shrilly when we removed its thorns from his coat.

Narrow-waisted, large-chested, tiny Pretzel trots like a pony, his paws barely touching the ground. Body erect, back arched, head up, nose forward, he walks with his tail standing high and curving over his back. His mouth remains partially open, his pink tongue protruding slightly.

"Cute."

"Cute."

"Cute."

That's what people say, and how puppy-like he appears as he ascends Camelback Mountain. He evokes smiles in people he passes.

W-A-L-K-Ing Laps In Luxury

Chic, gracefully-quick, Pretzel strides with Bailey and us along the paved bike paths running beside the streets of the Green Belt of Scottsdale, trots along canal paths, resort rows, playgrounds and golf courses. This area belongs to Pretzel. Cyclists, joggers, walkers, in-line skaters make way for him.

"How beautifully he walks!"

"Thank you."

"Gorgeous animal!"

"Thank you."

How excited Pretzel is to be in motion out in the open. His tail wags vigorously. This is his Lap of Luxury—the Sonoran desert blooming with lush, emerald green golf-courses paved with perpendicular lanes. This is where he struts. Only in the streets of Scottsdale does he take charge of Bailey, lead the expedition, and decide when it's time to sprint. Attached to both their leashes, we obey the dogs and go tearing after them.

On these walks, Pretzel possesses Bailey, too, making sure that Bailey has no canine friend other than him, and that he will remain severed from the Society of Dogs forever. He disallows Bailey the opportunity to befriend any we meet on the path. With undignified, high-pitched, illogical yelps of agony, and total overreaction, he embarrasses us when he forbids any well-meaning Canis Familiaris to sniff Bailey's or his own behind. His reactions set Bailey off on a tirade too, and the two badly-socialized South African hooligans disgrace us.

"Excuse them."

"Excuse them."

"Excuse us."

We apologize to dog owners who look at us as if we've crawled out of Gorgonzola. *Pretzel and Bailey are still Legal Aliens,* I wish to tell them. *South Africans, still. Mere holders of Green Cards, so please excuse them. By the time they qualify for citizenship, they will have mastered the way an American dog conducts himself while walking.*

South African dogs dominated sidewalks during apartheid. They had terrible attitudes. Attacked passers-by. Having been brought up in a society where many of the laws were difficult to respect, some dogs, like their owners, broke them.

"Now that the old laws in South Africa are obsolete, are people free to stroll the sidewalks, while dogs are gated?" A rhetorical question for N. While we walk, I ponder the meaning of freedom and walls.

Gone Missing

The gate to our garden is constantly closed so Bailey and Pretzel can't get to the sidewalk and street without us. We obey the leash laws of this country, and wonder how the dogs we had in South Africa survived into old age without them, particularly when the streets nearby were full of traffic, and the sidewalks patrolled by tyrannical dogs. Nothing more than good luck, probably.

A few days ago, Pretzel fled through the open garage door as I was helping a guest with many, heavy suitcases, move into the house. *Not another one of those,* he must have thought as he ran as fast as he could from the presence of yet another visitor claiming all his space in the house. We didn't notice his absence till hours later when we sat down to dinner.

"Where's Pretzel?" N asked. Bailey was jumping up and down on his hind legs demanding food, but Pretzel wasn't at his side.

"Pretzel? Oh my God, I haven't seen him!"

We looked in the bedroom, the dressing room, behind couches, inside, outside, everywhere. We called him. There was no response.

"He got out!"

"How?"

The only opportunity he had to leave the house was when we had transferred the luggage from the car to the guest room.

"Oh shit, how could I have not noticed him in the garage! Oh, no, I forgot to put his collar back on after his bath!" Little Pretzel, with no street smarts was on his own amid roads teeming with huge vehicles—Chevy Blazers and Nissan Pathfinders, Dodge Dakotas and Toyota Tacomas, all manner of big, vicious, egotistic gasgobblers, obliterating any view of a little, white, fluffy, terrified dog. "Oh God, what if he tries to cross Hayden Road!" We always cross it when we take them to the park.

Images of Pretzel, confused and frenzied, bolting headlong across Hayden flashed before my eyes. "He'll get killed!" Pretzel mangled, irretrievably entangled in the chassis of a pickup truck and lost forever from our view was too unbearable to contemplate. But it was a possibility. He could never, on his own, safely cross Hayden.

"Let's go! Quickly!" N and I, abandoning our guest, ran up our street to where it intersected with Hayden.

Vehicles continually whizzed by, but there was no sign of Pretzel. Not in the street, not on the sidewalks, not in the park or around the lake, not in the bushes or the surrounding neighborhood. Coyotes sometimes wander in the wash. Eagles and hawks fly overhead. Could he have been eaten?

Little Pretzel, lost most of the time in his own confusing, internal world, habitually unable to comprehend his needs and motives, his very canineness, Malteseness, and his foreigness, couldn't possibly know where to go or which was his path home. He'd never been away from home alone. He'd never been alone. If we weren't in the house, Bailey was.

I have been lost many times in my life because of an innate directional inability—or perhaps because as I drive, I dream and fail to observe or make a mental note of where I've come from or where I should be going. Getting back is often challenging, so I empathized with Pretzel. His choices were confounding—dangerous streets, crossroads, dead-ends, washes, sidewalks, footpaths with toe-ramming, stepping stones leading up grassed embankments. How was he to know the right route home?

"He needs a haircut," I say to N. "Won't see through his bangs."

What a plight! Could Pretzel survive a desert-hot night when he is used to air-conditioning set at seventy-four degrees? Mentally, transcendentally, I willed instructions to him: *If you panic Pretzel, you'll never find your way home. Take a deep breath. Focus. Think.*

It was too late to call animal shelters. We couldn't help him.

Small, White Male Maltese Missing.
Please call.

We put these notices up on poles and mailboxes. But who would be out in the dark to read them? No one. We stayed up all night hoping to hear him scratch at the door—as if he'd ever done that before.

At seven a.m the next morning, we started calling the animal shelters or related, sometimes barely, institutions: the Arizona Humane Society, Exotic Animal Rescue (but Pretzel's not exotic), Animal Control, Animal Rights, Liberate Wildlife, the list went on. Few were open. So we paced the streets and called Pretzel's name, paced and called. At nine a.m., we started calling the shelters again. By one o'clock that afternoon, there was still no news. Our little dog was so, so lost. Would we ever see him again?

The phone rang late in the afternoon. An animal shelter. Someone had called them about a white Bichon male. Maybe they were wrong. Maybe it was a Maltese. I was given an address about five blocks away from where we lived and sped there muttering all the way: "Please, please, please let it be Pretzel."

A gray-haired woman drew up outside the house in her car at the same time as I did. Together we slammed our doors and walked down the garden path. Felt like a race. She carried a basket to the front door filled with soft, fluffy, baby blankets. She quickly rang the bell. Winner, it seemed, was the one who entered the house first. She did.

"I've brought you the basket, Emily," she said. Emily took it and looked at me coldly.

"I've come about the dog. Believe you called Valley Rescue. May I see him?"

"He's in the kitchen," she said. "I'll get him." She brought in Pretzel!

"Thank you. Thank you."

I was happy. He was happy. Both women looked unhappy. I realized that the basket had been prepared for Pretzel. "Where did you find him?" I asked.

They had rescued him from the corner of Hayden and Chaparral the previous afternoon. "We took him home and called the shelter today. We would have kept him if you hadn't come."

Batdog

Pretzel, we live in a global world. Dogs immigrate. No dog is an island. Kennels are connected. You are disconnected, so develop your associative skills. Improve your general knowledge. Broaden your horizons. Use your intelligence. I enjoy communicating with Pretzel because he is a listener. Doesn't talk much. Doesn't babble. Thoughtfully silent. Why do some people take so long to say so little? Dogs don't. Pretzel doesn't. *Do you know any dogs that yap on and on, Pretzel?*

This morning, just for fun, I devised a questionnaire to try to understand him better. Then promptly answered the questions I posed:

Q: Is Pretzel intelligent?

A: He has some abilities, some signs of intelligence.

Q: Is he adaptable?

A: No.

Q: Could he ever learn to transfer information from one situation to another and not be so afraid of the new?

A: I don't think so.

Q: Can he solve problems?

A: No.

Q: Does he display any form of advanced mental acuity?

A: I don't think so.

Q: Does he have inspirations?

A: No.

Q: Avocations?

A: No.

Q: Aspirations?

A: Yes—to be taken seriously by Bailey.

Q: Does he have predictive powers?

A: He predicts catastrophes all the time.

Q: Creative abilities?

A: Haven't noticed any.

Q: Oratory skills?

A: Barks monologically.

Q: Does he have mind-boggling illuminations?

A: No.

Q: Can he herd sheep?

A: They would herd him.

Q: Retrieve game?

A: They'd retrieve him.

Q: Assist the disabled?

A: Perhaps. When Bailey hurts himself, Pretzel compulsively licks him better.

Q: With a flask of brandy dangling from his neck, could Pretzel rescue people marooned on frozen alpine slopes?

A: Not likely.

Q: Can he sniff out bombs and bombers?

A: No, he's not that kind of dog. Couldn't be trained to do so.

Q: Could he ever learn to eat his food before Bailey does, before the birds do?

A: No.

Q: Could he ever learn to use the doggie door and conserve household energy?

A: No.

Pretzel scores low in this test. But sometimes we think we see sparks of intelligence in him, yet fail to positively identify an ability. Lights flicker uncertainly in Pretzel, and dim quickly. Do we try hard enough? Do we have low expectations of him and does this influence Pretzel's feelings of unworthiness? Could this lag in intelligence and the suppression of his potential result from Bailey's hierarchical system: *obey me or I'll sit on you; submit or I'll eat your supper?* Could the fact that Pretzel was thrust under Bailey's domination without any established persona of his own, at only four weeks old—not six weeks as the breeder had declared—contribute to his insecurities? At four weeks, he was too young to have learned much about his dogginess from interactions with his mother and siblings. At three-hundred-and-sixty-four weeks, he still hasn't learned enough.

And yet, Pretzel does have one area of real achievement: bodily intelligence. I love watching him move. We often call him *witblitz,* white lightning, because he is an exceptional runner. When he sprints around the house at breakneck speed after coming in from a walk, or celebrating our return from a day or evening out, he is euphoric. Jubilant. This is his performance. Some kind of echo-locating intelligence comes into play. However small the room, Pretzel receives back echos from the walls, chairs, and couches. Skids to a halt within centimeters of their surfaces, before he levitates again. Never collides. When he dashes around the house or jumps from chairs or the patio table, BATDOG PRETZEL always lands delicately on his four paws.

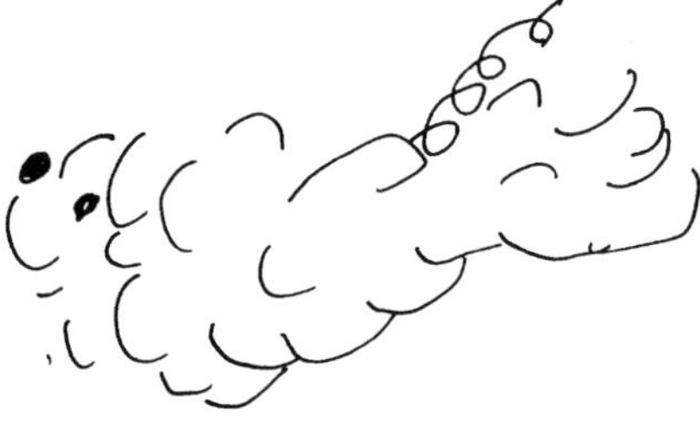

Identity Crisis

Last week, while waiting in the check-out line at Safeway, I saw Pretzel on the cover of *People Magazine*. There was no difference between the cover dog and Pretzel. They were identical—ginger ear, round, black eyes, upturned lips, big nose, curly coat, plumed tail. But the cover-dog was a Bichon Frise!

"Pretzel's not a Maltese!" I announced to N, showing him the photograph on the cover of the magazine I'd bought. "The camera never lies."

Ironic, really. Born in South Africa at a time when the government took pains to segregate people by placing them in racial categories entered into a national register, Pretzel was placed in the wrong one. Breed: Maltese it said on his pedigree certification, and so he was brought up to be what he wasn't. Reared to be like Bailey. It must have been disconcerting for him, a non-sporting dog, bred for hundreds of years to be a lapdog, to be expected to chase balls and participate in aquatic activities with an uncouth Maltese and a rugged Labrador. We had brought him up all wrong. Severed him from his Bichon-essence.

So what is a Bichon anyway? I went to the library: Pretzel's ancestry came from the Mediterranean area, sailed over rough and unknown seas with sailors who traded them for goods, for alcoholic beverages, for a variety of pleasures along the routes to the Philippine Islands, Cuba, Argentina, the Canary Islands, Tenerife, and Europe. Bichon Frises were once water dogs, descended from the water-wading, fowl-retrieving, Barbichons—small Water Spaniels, but they became lap-dogs, and Pretzel, obviously, had distanced himself from his watery past, memories he might not have wanted to recover. Could an ancestor, perhaps, have endured a near-drowning experience?

Hard to imagine Pretzel on the high seas tossed by powerful currents, battered by winds and almost drowned by massive waves at sea or tsunamis near the shore. Those images don't match him; others do: Pretzel, in a coronet and frilly collar, holding court in the royal houses of Spain, Italy, and France from his red, ecclesiastically and lushly embroidered-in-gold satin pillow, happily at ease with nobility and completely removed from the common, nautical dog of his origins.

Pretzel is a dog of the sixteenth century—adored, adorned and pampered. Bedecked with pompoms and rosettes, the Bichons of those times enhanced the appearances of their owners. Henry III carried his Bichons in a basket tied around his neck with ribbons, while the ladies of his court, using them as ornamentation, had their white, fluffy, cherubic canine faces peer out of the folds of their gowns and shawls. Pretzel, today, as I carry him over my shoulder, matches my white, non-designer-labeled tee-shirt while his white tail drapes over my faded, blue jeans.

Pretzel, the Bichon, needs to reassess his identity. We need to help him. How? I don't know. Apologize to him? *Pretzel, I'm sorry, sorry, sorry. I know you've been deprived of your essence. You've been what you're not for far too long. But many of us have been what we're not, also—and for far too long. Careless decisions, incompatible work, unenlightened assumptions. But we get over it. Make new choices. If we don't, we remain rooted to the wrong spot. We blunder in darkness and die without ever branching into secondary, tertiary—into multifaceted growth. We die without ever finding out who we really are. At least* ***you*** *know what you are: a Bichon and not a Maltese. Forget the past. Give yourself a second chance. Take charge of your salvation. Don't be a Dodo-dog, Pretzel. Learn to fly.*

I think about Pretzel's rescuer who had found him when he was lost in Scottsdale, and how she knew he was a Bichon when we didn't. Maybe she was saving him from more than a busy street—from the unfair expectations we had of him. *We'll stop encouraging you to wade in the lake, Pretzel, or cool yourself under the sprinklers. But you can't avoid water entirely just because you hate it. You still have to bathe every two weeks.*

I'm sorry, sorry, sorry, Pretzel. Too late for you to be thoroughly bred as a Bichon, when you've been outwardly reared as a Maltese. Who knows, with your looks, you might have been a show dog. Just look at your tail. Plumed perfection. Curves gracefully over your back. When extended, it's halfway to your withers. Powder puff coat. Plush to the touch.

Effortless trot. To win a prize, though, you would need a more cheerful attitude. But take comfort in your deviations from a standard: you're evolving into a new breed—into a Pretzel.

Questions for me to consider:

Q: Categories, labels, names, birthrights, insignias, emblems, species, breeds, genres, suborders, casts, persuasions—are these significant factors in the evolvement of a personality?

A: Their significance is based on the importance I attach to them.

Q: Could being mislabeled a Maltese have influenced Pretzel's emotional development?

A: If the label influenced me.

Q: Did it?

A: Yes.

Brought up to be what he wasn't, Pretzel had to leave his country of birth with its divinely, dogmatically-ordained belief in stratification according to origination, its uncompromising ban on irregular categories, its enforcement of complete segregation, and travel all the way to the United States to discover his roots on a popular, non-dogmatic, magazine cover.

Tumbling-Down Manor

After living in our house for five years, we're altering it radically, room by room, destroying much before we rebuild again. The hideous, elaborate, five-arm, wannabe-Waterford crystal chandelier which came with the house and dominated the dining room has been removed from the ceiling. I've offered the parts as dangling earrings—free—but had no takers. A relative, though, took the entire light fitting, and hung it on her outside patio. Looks funky in a rustic garden setting. Ugly mustard carpets and matching, oppressive valances and drapes—all inherited with the house—stand now in a container with other debris ready to be carted to a local dump.

Bailey enjoys it all. Each day of the two months we've been busy with the renovations, is different. There are new activities and sounds; this, for him, is fun. Life is interesting—a smorgasbord to sniff and chew. He attacks the ankles of the good-natured workers involved in the project, and they look guilty, as if they've done something to warrant his show of power. He tugs off (or perversely urinates on) the protective fabric or plastic sheeting which they have draped over our furniture.

Whatever the circumstances, whoever the contenders, he remains Top Dog by day and by night.

Wonderful, woolly, willful Bailey owns Pretzel, the house, and the space on our bed. He is Landlord of Tumbling-Down Manor by day. At night, he is Bedlord, the keeper of our toes. From his chosen position on top of the covers, he imprisons our feet and growls if we try to move them. We have to toss him up into the air if we wish to give our toes a respite—a stretch, a sprawl, a flow of lifeblood—but, quickly, Bailey lands on them again. *Gotcha!* We are his tenants with rights to lie under the covers, but not move while we sleep. And Pretzel, a mere squatter, Bailey's satellite and punching ball, is permitted to sleep only on the parts of our bedcover deemed appropriate by Bailey, and never on our toes.

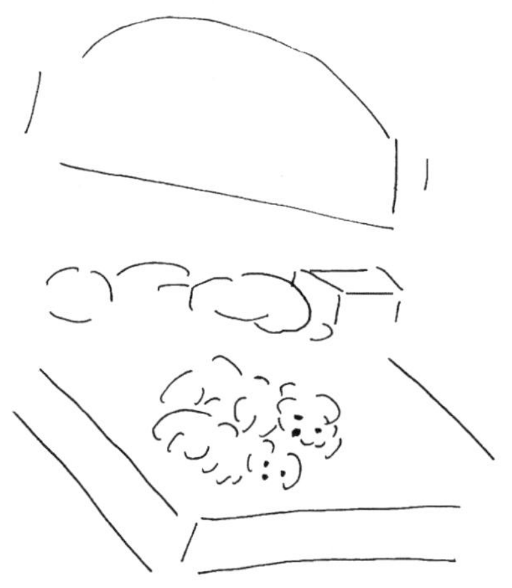

Each day, as the renovations continue, more layers of dust accumulate and descend. We sneeze and cough and wonder if we'll suffer any long term health problems. But it's exciting to watch a work in progress. One change suggests another and another. We improvise as we go along. Renovations, although time-consuming and messy, are fun.

But for Pretzel, May 14, the day the builders officially moved into our house and started their demolition, marks the beginning of a fast descent into a deep, dark well of bottled-up fears. These explode, one or many at a time, as his safe haven, inch by inch, is invaded and destroyed.

Booooooommmmm! Bannnnngggggggggg! That was the stud gun.

Pretzel's concerns grow in abundance. I can't keep track of them or predict what will scare him next now that he has moved firmly, fixedly, into his Age of High Anxiety—an agitated frame of mind and body which began the day we started renovating our house. To think that he once thought the flap of his doggie door was one of the scariest obstacles in his life! What he confronts now on a daily basis, is a reign of terror.

Immigration has already weakened Pretzel's faith in the ability of human beings to protect him against bogey-dogs and apparitions which he sees lurking in many corners, but on May 14, he completely lost his belief in N and me because we allowed electrically powered demolition, construction, assembly and installation tools to take over his space. We were no longer his saviors. We allowed the violent rumblings, turbulence, mass extinctions, and continuous bombardment from the builders. We allowed his world to implode.

We try to comfort him: "How's my little dog?"

"Nobody is going to hurt you."

"New walls are going to replace these crummy old ones."

We take him on a tour of the house: "See, these tools are harmless. That's only a bolt cutter. Those are needle-nose and bull-nose pliers. That's just a fire extinguisher."

We soothe him: pat, pat, stroke, stroke. Hugs—many of them. Carry him around with us. Give him lots of attention. Take him for walks. For drives. "Nothing to be frightened of, Pretzel. It'll soon be over."

Pretzel spends much of his time outside, despite the heat. He has dug a hole in the earth, deep enough to be moist. He wants to disappear into it and die. I keep going outside to find him, pick him up and embrace his sandy body, rigid yet quaking uncontrollably. He pants. His fur stands erect. He smells different. Of pungent fear. He is beyond comfort.

The high-pitched, caterwauling whines, thunderous claps, and piercing sounds of stud guns, high voltage cordless drills, and circular saws slicing fiercely through lumber, relentlessly send warning sirens through Pretzel's little body—all day long. While these offensive tools probe, screw, scrape, sand, and polish, Bailey blames Pretzel and lambasts him—not the machinery. He blames him for the orbit sanders which create lots of sawdust and make Bailey rasp and croak. He blames him for the jig saws which reverberate at three thousand strokes per minute, the sledgehammers which pound, the wire brushes which grate. He especially blames him for his headache.

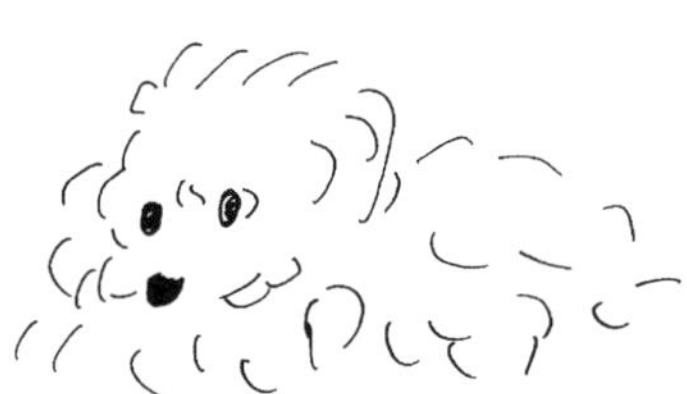

There Are Flies On Pretzel

Took about a year—felt much longer—but now our renovations are complete. Internal walls were removed and some replaced with smooth, curved, stucco ones. New kitchen and bathroom fittings supplant the old ones but all of these are constant reminders to Pretzel that powered enemies in the thousands, wanting to electrocute and slice him, once inhabited the house. Now, often, innocuous sounds evoke bad memories for him.

Bzzzzz is a bad vibration. The appearance of merely one fly informs him that all one-hundred-and-twenty-thousand-plus, tiny, aviating representatives of the *Species Diptera* will pay him a visit and buzz with as much electrical power as demolition equipment. Enemies continue to penetrate his refuge. He is still not safe within his own home. He daren't let down his guard.

"I can't help you, Pretzel. If you refuse to master the flap of the doggie door, how can I keep flies or mosquitos from coming through a permanent opening?"

Pretzel is tormented by flies. He spots them on the ceiling above him—wherever he happens to be. A mere whisper from one alerts him to where it hangs upside down with its suction-padded legs. Bobbing its body, it stares menacingly at him with its large compound eyes or it buzzes circles around him, its mouth extended, ready to land and bite into its food source.

"*Bzzzzzzz.* Gonna get you. Gonna get you. Rare Steak Bichon."

Perhaps empathy will help:

Pretzel, I too, have experienced the aggressive voraciousness of flies. I, too, know how painful their bites can be. My enemies were the Tsetse flies in the Okavango Swamps. Wait till one of them bites into you. Really dine on you. Suck your blood. Give you sleeping sickness.

I shudder as I begin to unpack the dishwasher. *They bit me, Pretzel, through my clothes with their ominously-protruding proboscises! Cunning, opportunistic creatures. Still hate them.*

These flies would penetrate the slightest opening of our car windows or doors, or follow our moving, four-wheel-drive jeep and pounce on us as soon as we stopped and ventured out. They were especially merciless each time the driver-of-the-moment (we took turns in driving) halted the vehicle. That's when they'd attack the rest of the group—sitting ducks on our flat-bottomed boat tied to the roof of the jeep for a better view of the game.

"Let's guzzle and gormandize! Cookout! Pig-out! Banquet!"

I became as paranoid as Pretzel, believing that these large, vicious creatures were especially attracted to me. And I was right. I learned later that Tsetse-flies have an affinity for dark colors such as the navy sweater and the blue jeans I wore. They bit through my thick clothing, inflicting wounds which were itchy and sore for weeks.

Pretzel, I understand your fear of flies. But you need to develop a sense of proportion. Not all flies are equal. Usually, their buzz is worse than their bite.

Pretzel doesn't react. Instead, he looks with aversion at a hairy house fly drowning in his milk.

Yuccckkkkk!

Last week, he had the same reaction to a Scottsdale sewer roach in the bowl of ground beef I'd left for him on our brick patio.

Yetttch!

I usually unpack the dishwasher quietly, so as not to disturb Pretzel, but I'm forgetting to do that now. Loudly I slam dishes on the counter.

Pretzel stares at me with a sense of foreboding.

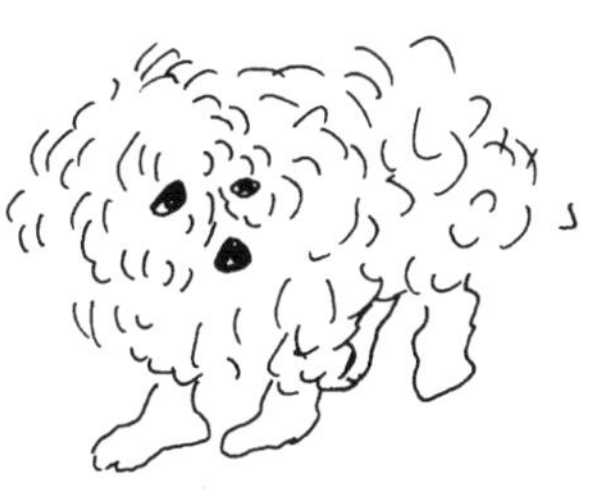

"Stop being scared of dishes, Pretzel. Flies, plates, cups, silverware—your fears are irrational. They go on and on. What do you think this meat platter is going to do to you?" With both hands, I hold it up above my head.

Smash! Crash! A commotion. How did it happen? I dropped the platter! Many pottery pieces scatter over the tiled kitchen floor. "Pretzel, wait!"

Pretzel, tail between his legs, bolts out of the open doggie door and into the garden where he frantically begins to dig a hole.

They're Coming To Get Me

Crockery, glassware, cutlery, pots and pans are now among Pretzel's greatest aversions. These weapons of assault, domestic beaker-bullets, pottery projectiles, air-to-Pretzel missiles, together with levitating insects, unnerve him. Rain, too. He runs for cover every time warmongering rain drops bombard him from the sky. His fears, these days, go on and on: the electric can opener, the singing kettle, the doorbell—so many, many things—a polyphobic dog under day-and-night attack. Don't know what to do with him.

Pretzel's phobias are time-consuming for me. Takes so long to pack or unpack the dishwasher. Merely lifting a plate off the kitchen counter suggests to him impending disaster: **Death by House Ware**. Opening the dishwasher heightens his fear-response, causing him to cower and flee to our clothes closet, or to dig deeper into his hole in the ground, his tomb under the orange and white bougainvillea vines.

How can anyone remove dishes from the dishwasher in complete silence? Even if Pretzel is in another room, he hears me, so I close him in our bedroom, and place towels in the space between the bottom of the door and the floor to ensure sound-proofing.

I try to recondition him. Carry him while caressing household utensils: "Nice, kind omelette pan," I say. "Cuddly ceramic cup." I open a cupboard door above the kitchen counter and sink. Show him the stacked shelves: "Our faithful Stonehenge Midwinter dinner service—a wedding gift we still use every day."

With a look of utter dread, he averts his face from the cupboard. His body droops. Life is scary. Fear sucks.

"You really puzzle me, Pretzel."

Not only do I worry now about his spiraling fears, but also the fact he has become so depressed. He is often withdrawn and reclusive. His body-movements have slowed. He slouches, skulks around the house with his back hunched, head down, refusing to observe anything but the ground. Occasionally, he looks at me, askance, his black eyes doleful, as if to ask whether I am aware of how sad he feels.

"I do understand how sad you are, Pretzel."

He then slouches even more, his body hanging so low that he looks like he might disappear into the floor. *Can't you see how worthless I am? Do you know how depressed I am? Do you have any idea of the burden I carry—the collective sufferings of my ancestors—those that were kicked, slugged, murdered, even eaten? Oh, my poor canis familiaris. I carry 100,000 years of collective sadness. I am the outcast dog, the peripheral dog roaming the outskirts of villages, being beaten and ignored, separated from my species, my mother, brothers and sisters. I am a Maltese with Bichon sensitivities, a Bichon with Maltese aspirations. I am dog dejectus, rejectus, perplexus. I'll always be scared. Disaster looms.*

"I know, Pretzel, and I don't know what to do for you."

Do you know that abandonment in early childhood predisposes infants for depression later in life?

"I've read that. Oh the problems you have...."

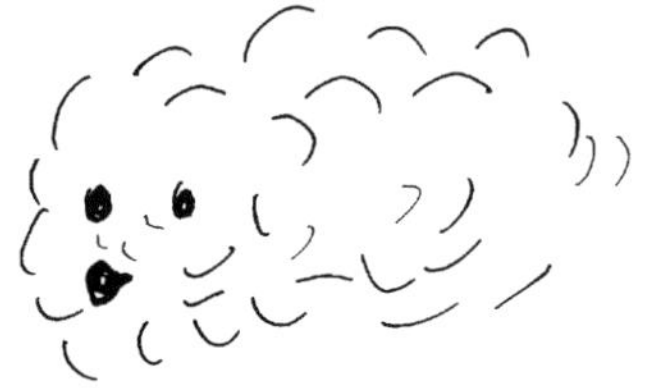

Life has become unbearably hard for Pretzel. Always highly-strung, our renovations have put him into a state of dread from which he cannot emerge. I can't let him suffer like this. I call the vet.

Questions For The Vet

"I think Pretzel has a mood disorder," I tell our vet. "He can't go on like this. He needs help."

"Okay, so what have you observed?"

"He's constantly terrified."

"Of what?"

And so I begin…

"I don't know why he's so frightened or what he anticipates. But he equates anything new with danger. Always expects the worst from a situation. He's a pessimist. His self-identity is confused. We brought him up as a Maltese instead of a Bichon. We deprived him overnight of chocolate to which he was addicted…"

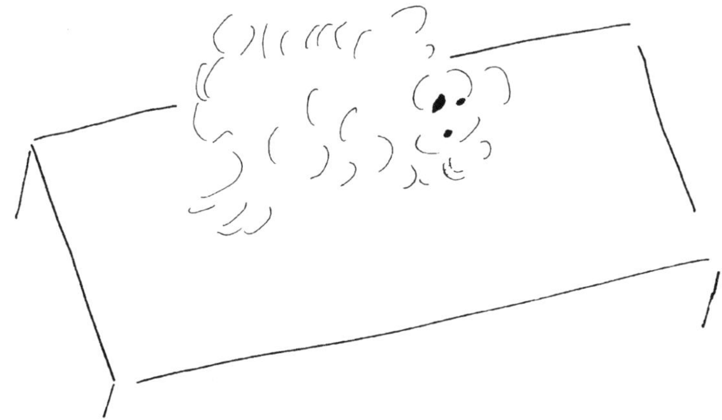

"Does he enjoy his food?" the vet interrupts.

"In a way and in many ways not." I think about Pretzel's attitude to food. Even the pleasure of eating is accompanied by a sense of loss, a feeling that the food will be snatched away from him at any time—like the chocolate. So instead of eating with relish, he eats with foreboding. Food, like life for him is bitter-sweet. Instead of enjoying its many aspects wholeheartedly, he feels an impending sense of its dematerialization.

"Problem-solving—how good is he at that?"

"Not good at all. He doesn't find his own solutions to problems. He also believes problems never go away. For example, ever since I dropped a plate in the kitchen, I can't stop him regarding crockery and cooking utensils as a major source of danger. I've tried to make him understand that they won't harm him. No, he's not a problem-solver."

Problems remain insurmountable for him. With Pretzel, they're permanent fixtures in his mind, solid walls that can't be moved. They're never forgotten. Once he has identified something as problematic, it's impossible to make him see it differently. He becomes lost in his obsessions, immune to any kind of reality check I can give him.

The vet talks into his dictaphone: "Mood disordered. Paranoid. Obsessional. Maladaptive personality type. Borderline psychotic? Yes, possibly."

"He is constantly aware of his vulnerability," I add. "He has low self-esteem. Maybe that's because Bailey has always bossed him and never let him feel competent. He has such raw emotions. It's sad how intensely he feels. We did some renovations on our house and he has never recovered from that. The memories keep intruding and I think he associates crockery with the noises of that time, with what he perceived as great danger. I think the house renovations were a deeply shocking experience for him—life-threatening, in fact."

"Does he startle easily?"

"Very." I think about how quickly acute distress overwhelms the coping mechanisms of his fragile body. He trembles and quivers at the slightest discordance or change in his environment. "I believe there are dog psychologists. Do you think he needs one?"

"No, that wouldn't help," the vet answers.

"I suppose not." What a psychotherapeutic task it would be to deal with Pretzel's psyche! He could never reach self-understanding. He needs a buffer against the rawness of his emotions.

"Pretzel needs Prozac,"says the vet.

Transformation

Pretzel sprang up from his sleep this morning. Horrified, he jumped off his duvet, placed in a corner of our bedroom, and ran around the room—round and round.

"Are you alright, Pretzel?" I knew he wasn't. "It must be the Prozac!"

Thursday, 7:15 am., two weeks after he had started his daily dose of Prozac, he was undergoing a transformation. I was his witness.

"Pretzel, what's going on?" He looked so different. I hadn't even noticed a subtle personality change in him since he'd started taking the drug, but now he was undoubtedly undergoing a heavy psychological disturbance.

"Something's happening to Pretzel!" I called to N who was in another room.

Pretzel ran frantically past N, then around the house, shaking his coat vigorously, trying to rid himself of whatever was attached to him.

"He doesn't run like Pretzel!" I shouted. "He looks peculiar. Something's moved into him!"

"What!"

"Just look at him. **Look at him!** He's not himself."

"Then who is he?"

A strange, invisible creature had commandeered Pretzel's little body. Not a second self—nothing like himself. Not a shadowy other. Not a doppelganger. An alien personality, intent on staging a complete takeover, was doing just that—infiltrating his psyche: *Gangway! Crash, bang, I'm moving in.*

"What should we do?"

"Let's watch Pretzel for a while," said N. "Try and gauge what's going on."

"Looks like he's possessed. Spooked." The Bogey-Dog that Pretzel had expected for so long had finally come. Invaded him while he slept, deeply, securely, innocently, on his vulnerable belly because he never (even after two weeks on Prozac) took the chance of exposing his soft underpart.

Then Pretzel began barking. High-pitched hysterical yelps. He darted around the house. *Out! Out! Out! Leave me alone!* Agitated, terrified, he hurtled into the sitting room, the kitchen, back to the bedroom, into the garden. It was obvious to me that he was doing battle with his altering state of consciousness, with an internal source of alien control. He was fighting for his life. Fighting. Fighting.

Please leave me alone, Pretzel beseeched. He couldn't reclaim his host body from the abductor, nor find a place to hide. Everywhere that Pretzel went, the intruder followed. And then, everywhere that Pretzel went, Bailey, sensing something was terribly wrong, followed, barking loudly. He chased after Pretzel as Pretzel ran away from himself. Bedlam!

"The vet!" we said.

"Need to straitjacket him," said N.

Leaving a barking Bailey on the patio, we restrained Pretzel in a bath towel, and rushed him to the vet.

"Something terrible is happening to Pretzel! Look at him." We unwrapped the poor dog.

Pretzel hurtled around the enclosed cubicle. He yelped. He howled.

"A psychopharmacological episode! We'll lower the dose of Prozac," said the vet.

Pretzel was tranquilized and by the time we arrived home, he was asleep. I carried him inside. He slept like a log on his duvet, but not the Bogey-Dog. Too calm inside for him. *Knock, knock, let me out.*

We never heard the Bogey-Dog go, but when Pretzel woke up later, he was gone, and Pretzel was calm.

Transformation Two

A few mornings later, Pretzel's second transformation occurred. It was early when he woke from a deep sleep at the same time as I did. He looked different—unusually calm and at ease with himself. In a light of white amid the floating rose blossoms of my imagination, Pretzel stood on a huge, open, white duvet-shell, his hair lifted by the breeze of the gentle god of controlled atmosphere. Air-Conditioner, himself, caressed Pretzel. The deep, dark, chaotic, churning anxiety of the past months, his intermittently noisy dreams, and his very bad psychopharmacological trip on Thursday, had been replaced by a Botticelli-like tranquility.

"The Birth of Pretzel," I said.

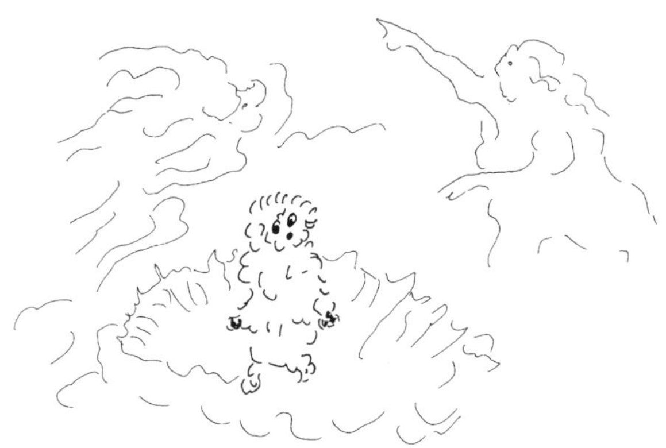

With his tail wagging, his neck thrust forward, his jaw tilted to the ceiling, his lips turned up, his little teeth exposed, Pretzel smiled at us. It was obvious that Prozac, the dose perfectly tailored to an eleven-pound dog, had miraculously altered him. Liberated him. Entirely changed his outlook on life and on his future. *Goodbye depression and panic attacks. Won't miss you at all. I'm happy, oh so happy…What a wonderful world!*

It's A Wonderful World

"Prozac has given Pretzel courage," says N. "Feels less oppressed."

"That's true. Yesterday he barked furiously at Bailey when he tried to take his food. Bailey actually moved away."

"No more signs of depression."

"More energy."

"Eats with relish. You know, I can empty the dish-washer in his presence without seeing that look of foreboding cross his face. Doesn't even leave the kitchen any more. I think that now when faced with problems, he's capable of finding solutions."

"But not with the doggie door."

"No, it will always have to remain open."

Yes, thanks to a mood-altering drug, a new dog has been born and Pretzel is back to the halcyon days of his Johannesburg past—to fine tranquil moods, enhanced now by glorious, sun-bright, Prozac colors. Blazing, electric, Kingfisher blues, greens, purples, and oranges illuminate his world as he cavorts with Bailey in our back garden—barking and sprinting. They race each other, coming to skidding halts just short of a wall, a tree, or a nose bump.

Prozac has assuaged his fears, improved his self-image. Given him a life. He is resilient, chirpy, less shy, not scared any more. Definitely more assertive. N and I are thrilled. We marvel at the transformation and tell each other and whoever is interested—or not—all about it.

"A wonder drug!"

"A new dog."

Every day, Pretzel invites us to play. *Chase me. Chase me.* His body is ready to pounce. To bolt. With his front legs stretched forward, his face lower than his shoulders, his rear end up, he is crouched and cranked to run. He looks up at us expectantly: *Well guys, are you prepared for a walk? A sprint? A race? What's taking so long?*

"We're ready."

When we return from our thirty-minute expedition, he joyfully reunites with his duvet on the floor of our dressing room, as if he had been parted from it for years. Seeing it anew, he jumps on it, rolls on his back and wriggles from side to side, sensuously enveloping himself in the texture, fragrance and softness of the fabric in the same way he does when he discovers a heap of raked vegetation in the corner of the garden or manure on the grass next to the sidewalk.

Pretzel's been on Prozac for a few months. He's reborn.

It's For My Dog

Hate picking up Pretzel's Prozac from the pharmacy. "It's for my dog," I always say when I call in.

"It's for my dog," I say again when I pick it up, countering the bad habit of one of the employees who calls the customer's last name loudly (Pretzel goes by our family name) and announce the full title of the prescription medication when it's ready for pick-up. The depot is located against the back wall of our busy, local supermarket, right next to the milk and eggs.

Today, what I feared finally happened: "Has Prozac helped you?" a woman asked me.

"It's for my dog but he's much better now," I tell her. "He'd been suffering from post traumatic stress syndrome, and this further exacerbated his existing mood disorders—depression as well as obsessive-compulsive disorder."

"Oh," was her response.

"He doesn't make enough serotonin on his own. It's a neurotransmitter thing. Prozac increases brain-serotonin transmission."

She quickly heads in the opposite direction.

"You should try it yourself," I call after her.

Not only have I found it uncomfortable picking up Pretzel's medication, but it hasn't been easy administering it to him. We give it to him in liquid form and he thinks it tastes disgusting. Vile. He screws up his mouth: *No way, no way. I won't take it.*

"Can't be **that** bad, Pretzel." I chase him around the house until I finally corner him, hold his face and nose, and eventually force it down his throat.

Yuccccckkkkkkk. Shudders run down his spine.

"So, it is that bad." I can't bring myself to taste it. Not sure what it might do to me. Make me into a happy dog. I've tried hiding it in his food but to no avail. Like the fairy tale princess in *The Princess and the Pea*, Pretzel can still detect a speck of Prozac hidden under many layers of food.

I call the vet: "Almost impossible to get Prozac down Pretzel. I dread giving it to him every morning."

The vet gives me the name of a pharmacist who creates designer Prozac for dogs. I'm hopeful he won't call our name out loudly when he dispenses the medication.

"I disguise it with meat," the designer pharmacist tells me. "I can keep changing the ingredients until we find what he likes. Lamb, beef, chicken."

He is discreet when he dispenses the drug, but the exercise proves costly, and none of the experiments work. There's no disguising Prozac. It's *yucuccccccckkkkkkkkk!!!*

I give up and deliver it to Pretzel in the unpalatable liquid form in which it had originally been prescribed. *Yuccccccckkkkkkkkkkkkkk!!! Yucccccccckkkkkkkkkkkkkkk!!! Yuccccccccccccckkkkkkkkkkkkkkkkkk!!!*

"Time for Prozac, Pretzel." Every morning, I chase him around the house, catch him and then with an eye-dropper, shove the liquid drug down his throat. "Say thank you to Prozac. It's doing wonders for you." But I worry that the daily struggle might counteract the beneficial effects of the drug.

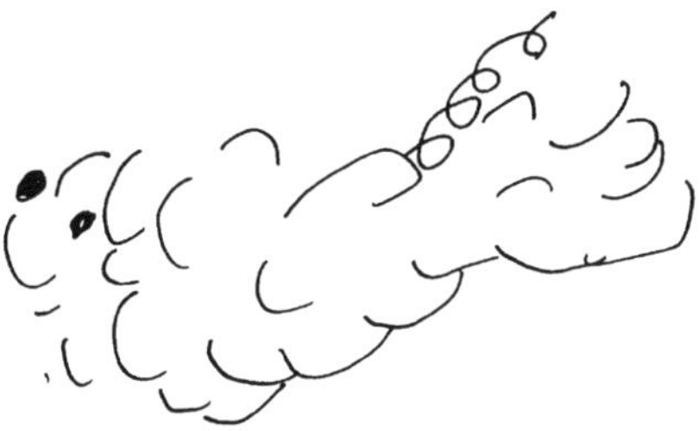

Citizens Canines

First came the interview for citizenship. We answered questions about the United States—from information in a booklet we'd diligently read in advance: "What color are the stars on our flag?" White. "What are the 49th and 50th states of the Union?" Hawaii and Alaska. "Whose rights are guaranteed by the Constitution and the Bill of Rights?" Everyone's. Pretzel's and Bailey's, too? There were more questions. We knew the answers. Then. We'd forgotten some by the time the swearing-in ceremony took place a few months later. Yesterday.

We are now citizens of the United States—seven years after first coming here. Our little dogs, twelve years old now, are Americans, too. Senior citizens.

"Congratulations, both of you."

Like us, they have fully absorbed the essence of being American—freedom, magnanimity, ambition, optimism, self-examination, re-creation, shopping at Costco. Eating jerky.

The swearing-in ceremony was moving. About a hundred people became citizens together with us. Volunteers were requested to speak about the personal meaning of the event. I thought I'd like to discuss what becoming an American meant to me while throwing in some anecdotes from my past. When I heard the contributions of some of the others: escape from oppression, from prison, torture, years of insecurity, I decided to remain silent. Being chased by hippo and elephant while exploring the wilds hardly seemed worth recounting.

We're all citizens now! We've changed. Matured. A result of new challenges. Much stimulation. Pretzel and Bailey are less antagonistic to other dogs when they meet them on the street. Probably understand that they now live in a big pond, and there's enough opportunities for all. Well-behaved dogs they've seen around the lake or on television have served as role models. Pretzel's and Bailey's behavior is much improved.

Physically, they're doing well. Their teeth are white (frequently visit the vet for dental treatment, cleaning and root canal work), their diets are balanced, and they are toned and fit. Psychologically, they've grown according to their potential, and lack of it. While Bailey transcends boundaries, Pretzel seeks them. Both are law-abiding. Respect the rules of the Home Owners' Association. Bark less frequently at night. Deserve their citizenship.

The United States is most definitely Bailey's milieu. He's a self-made dog. Self-challenging. Believes in self-improvement. Confused, though, about doing-the-right-thing and doing-his-own-thing. Generally, opts for the latter. Bailey thrives in his new country. Accustomed to self-aggrandizement, he now thinks he is a Rottweiler. Never cowers when a big, powerfully-built dog confronts him.

Pretzel has finally adjusted, too. Will always have many fears, but he is chirpy, garrulous, smiles frequently—a happy-barker. He is more optimistic. What has changed him? Prozac—certainly. America? Perhaps.

America alters us in small ways, too. Speech? Sometimes. Now, we say "tomayto" instead of "tomahto," "twenny" instead of "twenty." "Yeah" instead of "yes." I sometimes think I hear subtle linguistic modifications in the dogs, too, in the sound of their barks, for instance, which seem more nasal.

Old Dogs

Today is hot. One hundred and fifteen degrees! Too hot to climb Camelback. June. So what do I expect? Moderate temperatures? A Johannesburg midsummer day—eighty-five degrees under a southern hemisphere sun would be nice. Strong winds in the late afternoon. Black sky. Flashes of lightning. A thunderstorm. Loud. Hail on tin roof. More sunshine. Cool evening. Need a sweater. Nostalgia setting in?

What does a breeze feel like? Can't remember. And rain? Waiting for rain. Forgotten the sensation of refreshing aqua-drops falling from the sky. Tickles on my shoulders, sparkling bubbles on my cheeks. Need a margarita. Annual monsoons arrive in July. Waiting.

Our hot little dogs spend most of their time inside. Burn their paws out of doors. They lie directly on the cool, tile floor. Cushions and duvets are too warm. Ten years-worth of Phoenix sunshine in their curriculum vitae—about three thousand days. We even endured a daytime temperature of 122 degrees!

Pretzel and Bailey have grown old. Two little geriatrics on heart medication, two intrepid citizens, ignore the encroaching disabilities extorted from them for their fifteen years on earth. Pretzel pays less for his longevity than Bailey. Is in better physical condition. Has become the eyes and ears, the pilot-fish, the fact and destination finder, and guide dog of the deaf-and-almost-blind Bailey.

Poor Bailey is Pretzel's satellite. Follows him everywhere but at the same time bullies him. *So there you are. Your fault! Your fault! Don't you know where you're going?* Bailey's nose, the only sense on which he can still depend, smells-out Pretzel's whereabouts.

Years of comfortable cohabitation have progressed to a new symbiosis based on Bailey's present needs.

An escort—Pretzel provides the service. Comfort when in pain—Pretzel lick-lick-licks away open wounds, arthritic cramps, and congested coughs.

Protection—Pretzel tolerates no creature that would even think of harming Bailey as we walk around the lake, let alone a dog he suspects of waging war on an unsuspecting, blind Maltese. *Cowards! Wimps! Stabbers-in-the-back!*

Bailey is secure and can depend on his protector, healer, and chaperon. Side by side the two dogs walk, run or sleep. A Pretzel-On-Prozac reality has now become Bailey's own.

Where does Pretzel's goodness come from? I don't know. No commandments hanging on the walls of his life. No organized doggie congregation instructing him on compassion, on knowing right from wrong. No hell or damnation faces him for his lack of belief in a cosmic determinism. Pretzel is simply, naturally good.

To Be Or Not To Be?

To be or not to be on Prozac? That's our question. Does Pretzel still have to counteract anxiety? Depression? Obsession? Fear? Does he still need Prozac? Do flies still mutate and platters annihilate in his world view? Does he still have to dive for cover into holes he has dug in the garden when old enemies appear? We don't think so. Haven't noticed him becoming distressed lately when I'm at the dishwasher. Think that because his senses are dimming—hearing waning, cataracts clouding vision—his previous anxieties are now muted.

He's a happy dog. Demonstrates responsibility. Continues to take good care of an increasingly dependent Bailey. The going-blind leading the blind. What is Pretzel really like as a sixteen-year old dog? Perhaps, to find out, we should take him off Prozac.

Pretzel, you can't possibly still remember with clarity the renovations of the house or regard electrical noises as life-threatening events. You can't possibly still feel that disaster is imminent because someone has moved into the guest room. No, I think you've become a serene dog, and past fears, like your youth, are mere trace memories, diluted, never to be reinvigorated. You have grown old. Some advantages in that. An eclipsing effect. Time to take you off Prozac, Pretzel. Five years on a psychotropic, mood-enhancing drug is enough.

Liberation

Pretzel has been off Prozac for a few months. Doesn't need it. He remains happy. No doubt, encroaching deafness and impairment of sight have become substitutes for the medication, and a buffer against his feelings of hopelessness and fear. He's a joyful dog. Life is really nice now that he feels it through a haze of age.

And what a runner! Still! White lightning. Age has barely slowed him. Bailey can't keep up with Pretzel, and we battle to keep his pace. As Pretzel runs, his paws hardly touch the ground. Free as a bird. Free of Prozac. Free to be the old dog he really is.

I'm happy, oh so happy, …hear no evil; see no evil. What a wonderful world!

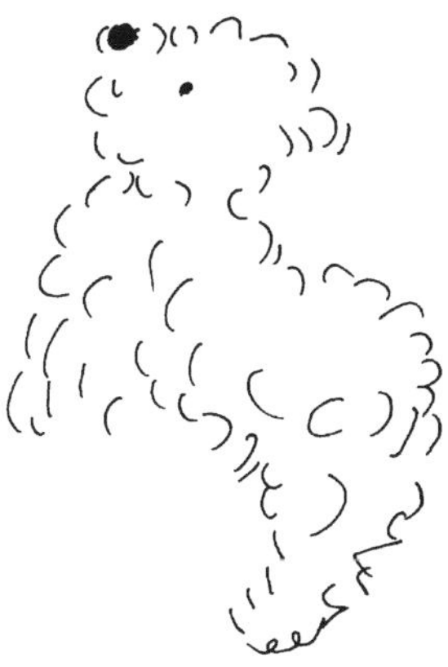

Hummingbird

We arrive home to find a hummingbird flapping frantically against the skylights.

"There's a hummingbird in the living room!" I shout to N, who is still in the garage. "Must have entered through the doggie door."

With feather-brained tropism, it sees only one route to freedom—the skylights. Knocks its head against it again and again. Becomes dizzy with delusion.

I have no idea how long it's been inside. Can imagine the confused state of its mind. Little thing, with a body weight of less than a penny, flies backwards, forwards, sideways, hovers, beating its wings rapidly, and flashing iridescent colors of emerald and ruby red.

Before opening the front door in the hope that the bird will fly out, I check on the dogs. Don't want them to wander off. They're asleep in our dressing room, unaware of the bird's plight. I feel sad. Two old dogs, between them seeing little and hearing even less, are increasingly unaware of their surroundings, of life in general, and today, of a hummingbird's desperate struggle for survival. Last night had been particularly bad for Bailey. He battled to breathe; fluid in his lungs. Medication helped a little, but we had to prop him up with cushions. Neither the dogs nor we had much sleep. Nor on other nights. Pretzel and Bailey make up for it during the day.

I cover the windows in the sitting and dining rooms with towels, hoping the hummingbird will be attracted to the light coming from the open front door, and fly out. "Please be more intelligent than other birds that have entered our house, and find your way out," I urge. "Please *notice* the open door."

It doesn't. "Hope it's lucky to have a hummingbird in the house."

I like to think it's lucky to have birds enter our house. I ignore superstitions stating otherwise:

If a bird enters a house through a window, bad luck will be the fate of the first person who sees it. (I'm usually the first person to see it.) If it enters through a door, bad luck is in store—unless the bird departs again through the same entrance. Yet, if a bird defecates on you from a dizzy height—you'll have immensely good luck. (No bird has ever defecated on me. Still waiting.)

"Hummingbird, hummingbird, fly away home." I will it to leave. Instead, it remains fixated on the skylights which I know we will now have to screen to shut out the light attracting the bird.

"The bird's expending too much energy," I say to N, as he enters the living room. "Could have been here for hours. Heart must be beating so rapidly."

"Probably in a state of torpor," says N. "Their body temperature drops. Heartbeat slows."

"Could be. Looks like it's in a trance."

"I'll get the stepladder and get on the roof," says N. That's the routine when birds fly in and can't get out. This one is no different from the other visitors.

"Here are the sheets." I hand him the navy ones we always use to cover the skylights. They effectively block out all light. "The problems Pretzel causes us because of the open doggie door. If only the bird would see the open *front* door and stop focusing on what's above."

In a Navajo legend, a hummingbird was sent up to see what was above the blue sky. It turned out to be absolutely nothing.

Be brave, little hummingbird. Don't die. N is going to help you. There are many myths about hummingbirds. They're said to be able to roll with the punches. Said to migrate on the backs of geese and other big birds. The Aztecs believed that hummingbirds were reincarnations of brave warriors killed in battle.

I see N's bearded face against the skylight as he starts to cover it with a sheet. The little hummingbird, intent on regaining its freedom, sees it, too. *Is it a bear? A dog?* The bird faints, instantly, on the ledge.

I run outside to call N. "Bring in the ladder. I think it's had a heart attack!"

N now climbs to the skylights from inside the living room. Places the cold, lifeless bird in the palm of his hand.

"Dead?" I ask.

N takes it outside and it immediately flies from his hand upwards into the fresh, clear air.

"Incredible," I say. "Was sure it was dead."

High up in the Andes of South America, the hummingbird symbolizes resurrection because on cold winter nights it appears to die but comes back to life during sunrise.

"I know there's a scientific explanation to all this, " I say, "but I feel we've witnessed a miracle." I shut the front door. The dogs haven't stirred.

Sick Bailey

Bailey is gravely ill: Heart failure. Lung congestion. But he is not ready to die. Bailey the Invincible fights death. A few times a day, he staggers stiffly to his bowl of food on the terrace and eats with surprising enthusiasm. Either the consumption of food remains enjoyable, or he knows it will maintain his strength and gain him additional time on earth. We observe him carefully. Don't want him to suffer. There still seems to be some quality to his life, even though he sleeps most of the time.

Pretzel, a self-appointed nurse, grows more obsessed with Bailey's well-being. Licks him endlessly. Lick-lick. Heal-heal. Is always at his side. How will he manage without Bailey? I'm not sure that he will. Sixteen years together is a long time.

We walk them both every night. Pretzel still walks well. Trots. Is nimble. He first accompanies Bailey on *his* walk, then later, has his own longer one with us.

"Let's go for a walk." The two deaf dogs don't hear these words anymore, but, instinctively know when it is time. Head for the front door. Wait.

We begin the first of the evening walks: Bailey drags his body past a few houses to the end of our block, where, with interest and focus, he and Pretzel, smell the daily news on the telephone pole. For more than two-thirds of their lives, they have stopped here each night, and like most readers, focused on what affects them directly. Bailey and Pretzel absorb piddle-printed stories by other reporters that work the beat—articles of dog interest that appeal to their emotions. They effluviate their replies: *overwritten ... superfluous ... narcissistic ... no news value ... agendarized ... not objective ... can't be trusted ... check your sources ... I smell more to this story—gonna chase it!* Pretzel runs ahead. Bailey tries to increase his speed. Can't. Difficult for us to coordinate the different paces of these leashed dogs.

Much has happened during their lifetimes in the country from which they emigrated, and the country in which they are now citizens. These apolitical dogs would not be aware of major changes in the South Africa they left behind—Nelson Mandela, released from prison and later sworn in as president after the first, non-racial, democratic elections. A new South Africa. Much has happened to the United States. Happiness, still pursued, is now clouded by palpable fear. Readers take note of terrorism and war—and the ominous warnings of more to come. A new America. An increasingly dangerous world. Count-down time? What's to be done? Who knows what the future holds as we continue with our everyday lives? Tonight, again, we'll try to make Bailey as comfortable as possible. For how much longer?

The Sounds Of Grief

We took Bailey to the vet last week for observation. We weren't sure if keeping him alive on medication was the right thing to do any more.

"We'll monitor him," the vet said. "Will call you in the afternoon."

"See you later, Bailey." I looked deeply into his eyes, clouded by cataracts.

He looked back at me, gravely, profoundly, as if to say, "This is it. The end has come."

That was the last time we saw him alive. The vet called a few hours later.

"Bailey had a heart attack on the examination table. I'm so sorry. There was nothing we could do for him."

Bailey had made the decision for himself. For us. Spared us the agony of passing a death sentence on him. Even though we'd known his end was near, we hadn't thought it would be that day. Life without Bailey. Hard to contemplate.

How light Bailey was in my arms when I carried him that morning to the vet for the last time. I felt his old age in the curvature of his spine, his withered, flaccid muscles; weak, wearying legs which could no longer walk him to the vet—just a couple of blocks from our house, or allow him to stand for even a short time.

How I miss Bailey. Feel his presence—the weight of his once solid, squat, young body. Thinking about his audacious insubordination makes me smile. Hooligan dog with an attitude, ready for a brawl. At the same time, loving, intelligent, amusing.

I feel his youth, his coiled energy rearing to charge around the house and garden. Enter any knockout competition. Win, of course.

A photograph of Bailey is now on the screen saver of our computer. I see it every day when I sit down to work. Dogs and cats live on in us but do they live on in dogs and cats?

It took about four days for Pretzel to realize that Bailey was not coming back, that he was on his own. So alone. No longer on Prozac, without a buffer against grief, he howled—raw, sore sounds. I rushed into the bedroom, found him standing at the doggie door—a little, white, round, fluffy ball in a rectangular room which looked so big and tall. So cold. I picked him up.

"Pretzel, what is it? Terror at being alone?"

Sounds deep with grief, despair, aloneness, abandonment, vociferated from his little body. Lamentations I'd heard before, but not from him. They come from a place rarely accessed. Primordial sounds that go beyond self. They reminded me of my own at my sister's funeral. Where did they come from? What are the sounds of grief?

"Pretzel, I'm here. You will learn to live without Bailey."

Our Lives Intertwine

Have a virus. And a fever. Am lying down in the afternoon. Never do that. Seems like such a waste of time. Nights are for sleeping. But I've joined old Pretzel in my bedroom today where he sleeps—for hours at a time—as life outside him hurtles by. Days, nights, weeks, months flash by. Flashback. How connected I feel to my past. To him. And how sad.

Sleeping in the afternoons, or even resting on a bed makes me think of illness, of my mother dying, my sister dying. Painful deaths. Melancholic memories of the past. And Pretzel sleeps on and on and on—in the mornings, in the afternoons, in the evenings—his rehearsal for death.

I watch him sleep. He is active, not passive. He seems closer to death lately, perhaps, but I can see that in his darkness, there are comfortable internal rhythms and though his life is no longer regulated by light and darkness, he is experiencing various states of consciousness. There *is* cerebral activity. I think I see him smile. *Tell me about your dream stories, Pretzel. They're pretty noisy. Do you have dreams of flying?*

He sleeps sprawled out. I pick him up, wake him, put him on my bed, look into his eyes. Love staring into his eyes, into his round, black pupils, trying to fathom his thoughts. He usually stares back but averts his head when he has had enough. Today, he looks into my eyes. *What are you thinking?* I ask him. *How can I ever understand your thoughts, your mind?* To some extent I can. I know when he is hungry, fearful, deliriously happy, but I wish I knew more.

How intertwined my life is with Pretzel's. We have lived together for so long. He is an immigrant dog, witness to our immigration, to the houses we lived in, to our emotions. To our dreams. As his synapses depart without a trace, he has fewer worries. He is quite serene these days. He is only in the company of humans. Doesn't seem to miss dogs at all. Has stopped looking for Bailey. In a way he has stepped into Bailey's shoes. Now he is Top Dog.

Dog Bondage

Pretzel hasn't walked well for weeks. His arthritis is bad. His steps have become shorter. No rhythm to his gait. No stride. He walks a few yards and has to stop.

"No stretchability—not sure if it's fair to walk him anymore," I say to N.

"Perhaps he needs stronger medication for his arthritis," says N.

What Pretzel also needs—badly—is a haircut. Bangs obscure his eyes again, although we cut them regularly. He is almost blind. Nothing should blur the little bit of vision he has left. He urgently requires a major haircut. He is lost in a shaggy mass.

Chunk by chunk, N removes sections of Pretzel's thick, matted hair from his back, neck, and head as I dangle him upright like a puppet on our glass patio table, trying to prevent his legs from sliding, forwards, backwards, sideways.

"He'll feel a lot cooler now," I say. Day temperatures have reached triple digits. "Uncomfortable for him to be held up in this way. Let's give him a rest."

We put Pretzel down for a few minutes. He drinks some water. Then we place him on the table again. This time on his back. The cold glass top cools him. N proceeds to cut his hair.

"My God, just look at this!" N has made a terrible discovery. "Look at the hair under his armpits! Completely entangled."

"Look at his back legs!" I say. "Just as bad. No wonder he can't walk. All kinds of knots. It's like he's been sewn up. Actually woven. See, these are the weft threads; these are the warp ones."

To think that we'd diagnosed his inability to walk even a few yards as severe arthritis. Poor little, trusting, dependent, old dog had been in bondage for at least a month. How cruel we feel for waiting until summer to give him a haircut. How badly we slipped up.

Old Dog Still Walking

A dog sniffs Pretzel's behind as we walk around the lake. Pretzel doesn't swivel around to chide the dog, or yelp with indignation. Old dog, lost in his own world, is increasingly less attuned to the exterior world. Sad that he is now indifferent to his own and to other dogs' posteriors. He has forgotten most old memories. Can't form new ones. In the past, he would never have accepted such an indignity.

Pretzel is tired when we start to walk. Moves slowly, stiffly, sometimes unwillingly. Wants to sleep and sleep and sleep. But once he finds his rhythm, he accelerates, and a younger Pretzel emerges, one with a nose to the ground, inhaling exciting particles of evidence of the past and the present. Alert, tail wagging, he locks into an odor and follows it persistently until it disappears.

Sometimes, he looks at me askance, gauging if I'm ready to join him in further discarding his old self in an abandoned race home, his rite of celebration for an eighteen-year passage on earth.

"Hey, Pretzel, I can't keep up with you!"

He is a puppy again. Transformed into juvenescence, he sets the pace. Sprints ahead at full throttle, and I am out of breath.

"What a cute puppy."

A passerby thought he was a puppy! "He's eighteen years old," I shout back as I continue to dash after him. I'm proud of my little fellow. See Pretzel run. Slows down a little as we climb a grass knoll. Then speeds down it. *Watch me! Yippee!*

For a few minutes he is *witblitz*. Has voided old age. But then he has to stop. Little legs won't carry him any further. I pick him up and carry him home.

Pretzel, with heart failure and on managed care, does well. He is happy. The After-Prozac dog finds peace as the memories of what had once frightened him fade, and as he ceases to hear the terrifying sounds of life.

Flying Saucers

Crash! Smash! Shatter! More shatters. And more! I run into the kitchen. I am alone at home except for Pretzel, asleep on his duvet in the bedroom. "What's happening!" A cataclysmic event? Is it an earthquake?

There is total devastation in the kitchen. Cupboard doors above the sink have been flung open. The cupboard shelves, collapsed, are now steep, slippery slopes. Cups, plates, saucers slip onto each other and hurtle out of the cupboard. Some appear to voluntarily jump, hoping to survive. Others—fighter bombers—veer laterally while in the air and attack flying objects. Smash those which already have landed. Everything comes tumbling down. Mounds of debris. Shattered lives. A war zone.

"Need a ladder." I quickly check on Pretzel. Sleeping. Run to get a short ladder from the garage. Mount it as it sways unsteadily on piles of smashed china on the kitchen floor. Try to straighten the sloping shelves. Try to close the cupboard doors. Not possible. Can't stop the force of the revolution inside. Plates and bowls, cups and saucers continue to topple. Nosedive. Fracture each other on the hard, tile floor. The violence of the scene! The waste! No holds barred.

I realize it's my fault. All these years, I had a perfectly good dinner service. Stonehenge—a wedding gift, part of my old life, which had endured children, many guests, countless meals, hand-washing, zestful electric dish-washers, immigration, and moving houses. Had twelve of everything: meat plates, fish plates, bread plates, soup bowls, fruit bowls, big platters, casserole dishes, tea and coffee services. Only two broken cups in all these years. Loyal, serviceable crockery.

Disloyalty to the old country and crockery. I am guilty of that. Replaced my old life with the new so casually, when, on a whim, yesterday, I bought another complete dinner service. Modern. Stream-lined. Put it in the cup-board, next to and on top of the ancient Stonehenge inhabitants. Into **their** temple. A bit of a squeeze. Two dinner services. One cupboard. Two nations. One land. Insufficient space for both.

Which service would contain our food? Which would be the most admired? Which would dominate? Which would I serve? None. Stonehenge reaped revenge on my thoughtless switch from the past to the present. There is barely an unbroken dish left in the ruins of two complete dinner services.

"What a mess!" The aerial strikes are over. Every-thing is quiet in the aftermath. "I didn't need another set. Where do I begin? Oh, not my coffee machine as well!"

There must have been such stress in the cocooned hypocenter, that pressure had to be released. Communi-ties nearby also suffered terrible destruction. Not only the coffee machine, the sugar bowl, and the milk jug, but antique green bottles, a vase with flowers, and a juice extractor were knocked off the kitchen counter. Fortunate that the area was not more populated.

Had Pretzel, years ago, sensed the pent-up emotions of the dishes in our cupboard? Could his fears of the objects I had put in and taken out of the dishwasher everyday been founded to some extent? They did have the potential to cause catastrophic events. Even to kill Pretzel—perhaps me—had we been standing by the sink during this unnatural disaster. "Some headline it would make," I say to the broom as I sweep up the mess.

The Great Kitchen Quake: *Immigrants from South Africa killed in flying saucer attack.*

I think about the reactions of some people from the past who had voiced their displeasure when we said our farewells to South Africa:

"Where is your patriotism? This is the best country in the world."

"Joining the Chicken Run?"

"There are earthquakes in California and that's not so far from Arizona."

"How can you immigrate to a country with such a high crime rate?"

Now, feeling vindicated, they would say of us:

"We told them so. The United States is dangerous. You're not even secure in your own homes."

I told you so. If Pretzel had witnessed this disaster in the kitchen today, these might have been his words, too.

"I'm pleased you heard none of this, Pretzel." He is still fast asleep on his duvet. Old age has its compensations. So does loss of memory. His cupboard, once full of recollections, is becoming increasingly bare. His cognitive abilities have declined. He is disoriented, has little understanding of situations, and is uninterested in much around him, or the pursuits he once enjoyed. He is indifferent to what he once feared. Dishes are neutral. A non-issue. Bygones are gone.

Memories Vanish

I sometimes think that Pretzel has forgotten himself. Asks for less and less attention.

His days are sadly dull. Unaware of the external world, he sleeps, urinates, sleeps, defecates, sleeps, eats, stares at walls, gets stuck in corners, sleeps, sleeps, sleeps. He is less shy and fearful simply because he is less aware. His mood has gradually altered, but not from drugs this time. He has Canine Alzheimer's.

"Do you think there's still a quality to his life?" I ask N.

"He's not unhappy," says N.

"Do you think the effects of Alzheimer's equal those of Prozac? Mutes his raw feelings, his fears?" I ask.

Could Pretzel possibly have any concept of himself still left? Did he ever have a self-concept—an awareness of his dogginess while he lived in our human world? His consciousness has been shaped all this time by his interaction with us. He gets his cues from us. We must be his definition of his South African-American-Maltese-Bichon self. Would he know he is becoming old? Would he ever wonder why his legs are so stiff, why he sleeps so much, why the familiar has become strange? He probably has no idea that he is running out of time. Lucky dog, not to feel the anxiety of imminent death.

Yesterday a puppy, today a very senior citizen. Eighteen and a half years old. In dog years, about one hundred and thirty! I choose to adhere to my childhood belief that one human year equals seven dog ones.

"He's ancient," I say. "The vet says he's the oldest dog in his practice."

Pretzel can barely see and bumps into our patio furniture as he heads for his food. He ambles in a particular direction and then stops in his tracks as if he's trying to recall where he was going. His brain shrinks as memories vanish. Can't form new ones.

"He's so forgetful," I say. "How can we help him?"

"Needs a diary to remind him of what he's supposed to do," says N.

"But he hasn't forgotten how to run."

At night, because it is cool—relatively, we take him for a walk. His arthritic neck, back and legs straighten as we progress, and suddenly he is off, sprinting through the suburbs, leading by his leash. Running for his life. Running from death.

Voices In the Night

I remember being scolded by a neighbor when we first moved into our present house because Pretzel and Bailey barked loudly one night.

"What kind of people are you?" the neighbor shouted to us over the wall. "Renters, I expect."

"Ever sooooo sorry." In the most affected, superior, disdainful, colonial accent I could muster, I apologized for my dogs. "It's the sense of entitlement of the pedigreed, you see. They think they own the night."

One evening, a few weeks later, we passed this neighbor as we walked Pretzel and Bailey. He stood on the sidewalk behind a tree, smoking. N saw him; I didn't.

Suddenly, overcome with nostalgia, I said to N, "I smell Africa."

"That's dope," said N.

"Someone's smoking dope?" I asked. That's when I saw the neighbor hastily open his front gate and retreat into his house.

Marijuana—we called it dagga—pervaded the air during our lives in South Africa. Thought, as a child, it was the scent of the veldt. Now, I realize its sweet, charred, spicy pungency coalesced with the dry, dusty perfume of the bush. I wonder if second-hand smoke accounted for my happy childhood, or if the lack of second-hand smoke in Arizona, contributed to Pretzel's need for Prozac.

The neighbor never chided us again, and we tried our best not to let the dogs bark at night. Wasn't easy. Dogs bark, cats meow, frogs croak, and all manner of cacophonies—police sirens, wails, snores, and dissonant dreams—prevail in the dark.

As Pretzel and Bailey grew older, they barked less. Pretzel, very seldom. The last time we heard Pretzel bark was months ago in the middle of the night, about a year after Bailey had died.

"It's a cat eating his food," said N who went outside to see what had caused him to be so vocal.

He barked for quite a while in the high-pitched indignation of his youth. Hadn't heard him do this for so long.

"Brings back the past," I said. "Makes me sad."

We didn't try to stop him. The neighbor had moved out by then. Something so nostalgic about his bark in the dark. A familiar sound. Wondered if Pretzel heard it, and recognize it as his own. He barked louder and with more confidence as he resurrected vocal chords, flabby from disuse.

"Pretzel, enough!" Unable to modulate his bark, it was now a screech.

"Shut up!" That was from the new neighbor.

Deaf Pretzel stopped. The pitch of his voice had become so high that he ran out of voice—out of sound. Out of vigor. N picked him up and brought him inside.

"Well done, Pretzel! You've still got it in you. You just tell that cat off." We showered him with compliments.

He hasn't barked since.

A World Of Silence

The clues that Pretzel has Doggie Alzheimer's are all there: restlessness when awake, sleeping most of the day, getting lost and stuck in corners, inability to redirect himself, staring into space, and increasing lapses in housebreaking activity. Lack of awareness that these incidents have occurred. He paces up and down, up and down, making us nervous. Appears to be looking for something. For what? For what was? For himself?

Took him to the vet again:

"Pretzel mainly has two states: deep sleep and anxiety when awake," I say. "He has a terror of being alone. And CRS."

"CRS?"

"Yes. Can't Remember Shit."

"Pretzel has definite signs of age-related canine cognitive dysfunction syndrome," says the vet. "Try Anypril. Might help."

It has helped, I think. He seems a little more perky. Saw him wag his pink, balding tail at inanimate objects—the plastic boxes that enclose his living area now at the end of our bedroom, and only allow him to exit through the open doggie door because of his incontinence. Anticipates something nice, perhaps, as he exits to the patio, only to become lost again in his confusion. Stands staring into space. Has no idea what motivated him to go outside.

There are so few signs left of the Pretzel-dog we knew intimately. He wanders through the geriatric chapter of his life as another dog inhabiting what might as well be another planet. He doesn't dwell in the comfort of familiar spaces any more—not in his enclosure at the end of the bedroom, not on the patio, where chairs, tables, walls, doorways are no longer where they are supposed to be, and not in his own body and head, where **he** is supposed to be—but isn't. Plaque deposits around the neurons of his brain rob him of the memory of the dog he was, and the familiarity of the environment in which he once lived.

"He still seems to know us," N says.

"Still some quality to his life. He eats, but leaves more for the birds."

Pretzel is unaware of the birds perched on his bowls while he eats or drinks. Buried inside his food is his crushed heart medicine and the Anipryl to ward off the effects of his Canine Alzheimers. Wonder what effect these drugs have on the birds, and the cockroaches—giant ones—that feed on his food.

The birds in the bushes and grape vines which overhang our patio, watch Pretzel's every move. They alert each other when he appears on the patio because they know food will follow. A cactus wren seems particularly focused on Pretzel. Often peers through the doggie door to see if he's up. Has come into the house and dive-bombed him awake. Saw him try to peck Pretzel as he walked towards his food. Was Pretzel too slow for the bird? *Gobble some of it, old dog, so we can finish the rest.* Pretzel sits now on his haunches while he eats, as Bailey used to do when his legs were too weak to support him. Pretzel usually forgets that he is eating. Sometimes falls asleep at his bowl.

So what does the future hold for him? Nothing hopeful. The tragic disease of old age will progress through other areas of his brain, and he will continue to go bump into objects that weren't meant to be there—in the night and in the day—until he dies. One thing we know for certain is that although we don't want him to suffer, we also don't want to take the power of sentencing him to death. So we observe him, hoping he'll know when it's time for him to go. *Pretzel, please don't let us be the ones to decide when to end your life.*

Pretzel is silent most of the time. Occasionally a whimper conveys fear, loneliness, hunger or discomfort, especially when being bathed. When we rub his withered body with a warm, soft, bath towel, he groans with pleasure. He hears nothing. Little response to external stimuli. He lives in a world of silence. Except when he dreams.

Sounds Of Dreams

Pretzel wags his tail as he sleeps. "Hic-hic-hic." And again: "Hic-hic-hic." Nothing to do with his digestion. Awake, he is silent, but when he sleeps, I hear the sounds of his dreams—his responses to something he experiences. He whimpers. Is agitated. Moves his legs as if he were running. Things are happening. Action.

These sounds are a response to an internal stimulation. A story unfolding? *What are you dreaming about, Pretzel? Are* **you** *in your dream? Is there a plot? Images? Colors?* How alive is his brain? Is he still capable of producing entertaining dreams?

I wonder about what happens to the content of Pretzel's dreams as his neurons die away. With no excitement from the outside to provide him with visual and auditory material, does he still have *in*sight? How much information is still encoded within his memory? He appears more alive when asleep than when he is not.

What is more real to Pretzel, his dream life or his awake one? *Ever see any of us in your dreams, Pretzel?*

"Do you think it's fair to keep him alive?" I ask N.

We have discussed this so many times. We don't have an answer. Pretzel has so little quality left in his life. Is increasingly lost in his dreams, isolated from external sounds.

"Is it worth being alive to sleep most of the time?" N asks.

"I don't know. I don't think you dream when you're dead. If you still dream, then you're alive. "

Sleeping is different from death. Perhaps when Pretzel dreams, he disassociates from his stiff, exhausted old body. Journeys to beautiful places. Flies to the moon. Communicates with the other inhabitants of his fantasies. *Do you enjoy your dreams, Pretzel? If you do, it means your life still has some quality.*

I think that Pretzel's ability to still dream is important. That, and his deep sleep, might be a rehearsal for death which we shouldn't interrupt, and a preparation for recognizing death when it comes. Will he know when he is ready to die? Is he already in a state of dying?

Pretzel is too weak to go on walks, but he still eats. Has some appetite. He eats to sustain his dreams. He dreams, therefore he is alive. As long as he dreams, he'll be here tomorrow and tomorrow and tomorrow.

Each tomorrow, I wake up and check on him. Is he breathing? Yes, because his chest expands and contracts. "Well, hello Pretzel," I say. I'm grateful every morning when I find him still alive.

Prison

Marooned on his duvet, solitary, so alone, Pretzel lives in his enclosure—still that boxed-in area at the end of our bedroom from which he has access to the patio. We hate seeing him this way. Have to step over his prison walls to pat him. He is slipping away mentally.

A decent dog, Pretzel never bit anyone. Seldom bared his teeth. Always, at heart—even when shrieking embarrassingly because another dog had approached Bailey—a pacifist.

I stroke Pretzel. He is tangible, material, verifiable. He is alive, but not for much longer. Barely eats. Is experiencing severe pain in his abdomen. Tumbles over as he desperately tries to get at the source of his suffering. Nothing has shown up on x-rays. Nothing can be done to alleviate the discomfort. The vet says it's probably a result of his dementia. Real pain—though not really there.

We consulted with the vet again today. "I don't think you have a choice. It's time."

"You're right."

"We don't want to abandon him," I say.

"Can't let him suffer," says N.

The time has come for euthanasia. Tomorrow morning, but he's still here, today.

Release

N and I sit in the waiting room with Pretzel. We hug him. Drugged, because of his pain, he sleeps. These are the last few minutes we will be with him after twenty years together. I think about the final hours I spent with my sister.

"Just a throat irritant." Those were the last words she said to me as I sat next to her in the ambulance rushing her to hospital. She had explained her cough but not the theft of her young life. That night she was in a coma. A week later—dead.

Here today; gone tomorrow. She faced no theological certainty, no guarantees. She faced death as she had faced life, with courage, never blaming any deity or any one else for the tragedy of her illness. Images of the joyful, stimulating, and sorrowful moments we had together remain in me, a keeper of her memory. Where will those moments go when I die?

I think about how wondrous it always seems to me when I fly at night over foreign cities illuminated by electric lights and imagine the people living in these lands so different and far from mine, speaking extraordinary languages, leading ordinary lives. Sleeping alone or together in beds in rooms with ceilings and walls. Eating at tables.

Doing city and rural things. Working. Completing chores. Loving. Grieving. Dying. How ordinary life is, and at the same time, how extraordinary.

The vet calls us into the examination room. We look deeply into Pretzel's unseeing eyes for the last time. Look into his darkness. Hug him. Can't take care of him where he is going. Oh, let him be okay.

"Goodbye, Pretzel."

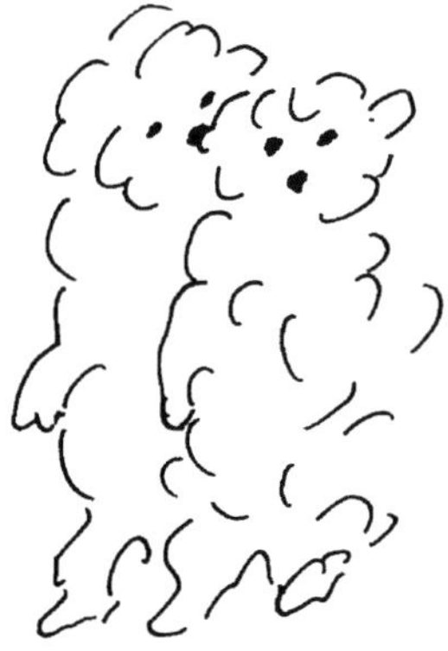

Where Is He?

We remove the doggie doors from the kitchen and bedroom. Too painful to look at them. We dismantle Pretzel's private abode, taking away the plastic boxes at the end of our bedroom and his duvet. The bedroom seems empty. Our lives, too.

A couple of days after Pretzel died, I hear a tap-tapping at the closed, glass doors of our bedroom. Insistent it is: *Tap-tap, tap-tap, tap-tap.*

"Pretzel! He is shut out of his room!" I know it can't be him but I run to the door.

The cactus wren stands on the patio, next to where the opening of the doggie door had been. *Why hasn't Pretzel woken up. Where is he?*

"I wish I knew," I say as I open a tin of Pretzel's food and give it to the wren—without the usual medications. Other birds gather. They eat up everything in the bowl. Slowly, I will wean them off doggie food.

Slowly, we'll learn to live without Pretzel. Here today, gone tomorrow. Life carries on, so we live, screening out the bad, focusing on the good, rearranging memories, filling our minds with comforting stories, seeking out in our dreams those who are long gone. We dream; therefore we are alive. We dream; therefore, we are.

A photograph of Pretzel, sitting beside Bailey, beams cheerfully at me on the screen saver of my computer. Whenever I sit down to work, now, I greet them both.

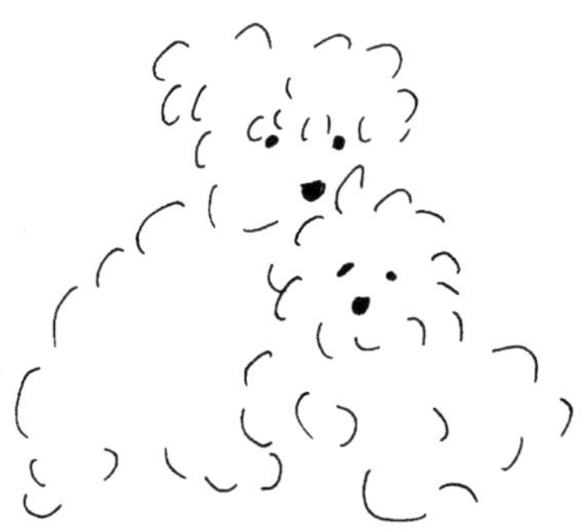

Made in the USA
Columbia, SC
26 November 2021